D1609289

EXPRESSIVE ARTS FOR THE VERY
DISABLED AND HANDICAPPED
FOR ALL AGES

ABOUT THE AUTHORS

Marilyn Wannamaker is a professional portrait painter, who has demonstrated and lectured on portraiture and oil painting throughout the mid-south region. She has shared her knowledge and enthusiasm for painting in numerous workshops, seminars, private classes and adult education programs, acquiring a reputation as an outstanding teacher of fine arts. In recent years, she has turned her attention to art therapy. Through post graduate courses in psychology at The University of Memphis and through graduate art therapy courses at The University of Illinois at Chicago, Wannamaker is researching and developing a foundation for integrating her experience as an artist with her belief and interest in applying arts and crafts to the healing process. Currently she is employed as an art therapist at The Guardian Foundation in Memphis, TN. Here Marilyn Wannamaker has experienced the profound effectiveness of art therapy as a means of working with clients who have suffered severe traumatic abuse. It is her sincere desire that this book be a helpful and positive tool for caregivers and their clients.

Jane G. Cohen, an award-winning artist, combined her dedication to the importance of art in our personal lives and her personal mission to make a positive difference in those who lives she touches to write and illustrate *Expressive Arts for the Very Disabled and Handicapped.* A successful insurance agent by profession, she has extensive training in business, estate, and pension analysis. Her articles have been published in professional journals, and her illustrations have appeared in "Project Calendar 1995," the 1994 fall issue of "Lifetimes," and *Crafts for the Very Disabled and Handicapped,* a full length book in rehabilitation therapy. She professionally illustrated a book of poetry, *Inside the Gates,* by Constance McDonald. Jane G. Cohen, a former Activities Coordinator and psychometrist, earned her Chartered Life Underwriter and Chartered Financial Consultant designations from The American College and bachelor of science in psychology from The University of Memphis. She studied drawing and painting at Memphis College of Art, The University of Memphis, and Ichiyo Japanese Art Center in Atlanta, Georgia. She lives with her husband Merlin Cohen, a stone sculptor, in Memphis, TN. They are the parents of five children.

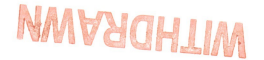

EXPRESSIVE ARTS FOR THE VERY DISABLED AND HANDICAPPED FOR ALL AGES

Second Edition

By

JANE G. COHEN

MARILYN WANNAMAKER

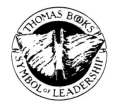

CHARLES C THOMAS • PUBLISHER, LTD.

Springfield • Illinois • U.S.A.

Published and Distributed Throughout the World by

CHARLES C THOMAS • PUBLISHER, LTD.
2600 South First Street
Springfield, Illinois 62794-9265

This book is protected by copyright. No part of
it may be reproduced in any manner without
written permission from the publisher.

© *1996 by* CHARLES C THOMAS • PUBLISHER, LTD.
ISBN 0-398-06704-X (paper)
Library of Congress Catalog Card Number: 96-23680

First Edition, 1977
Second Edition, 1996

With THOMAS BOOKS *careful attention is given to all details of manufacturing
and design. It is the Publisher's desire to present books that are satisfactory as to their
physical qualities and artistic possibilities and appropriate for their particular use.*
THOMAS BOOKS *will be true to those laws of quality that assure a good name
and good will.*

Printed in the United States of America
SC-R-3

Library of Congress Cataloging-in-Publication Data

Cohen, Jane G.
    Expressive arts for the very disabled and handicapped : for all
ages / by Jane G. Cohen, Marilyn Wannamaker. — 2nd ed.
        p.   cm.
    Originally published under title: Crafts for the very disabled and
handicapped. 1977.
    Includes bibliographical references.
    ISBN 0-398-06704-X (paper)
    1. Handicraft. 2. Handicapped—Recreation. 3. Art therapy.
I. Wannamaker, Marilyn. II. Cohen, Jane G. Crafts for the very
disabled and handicapped. III. Title.
TT157.K38   1996
615.8'5153—dc20   96-23680
                                                                        CIP

*TO ALL WHO USE EXPRESSIVE ARTS AND CRAFTS
THERAPEUTICALLY WITH THE VERY DISABLED
AND MENTALLY IMPAIRED*

Our thanks for coloring life with your art.

PREFACE

With this new edition, we have elected to expand the focus of the original *Crafts For The Very Disabled And Handicapped For All Ages*. Cognizant of current developments in crafts and other forms of art therapies, we have changed both the title and emphasis to encompass a broader range of the expressive arts.

The extremely disabled or handicapped person (who may or may not be institutionalized) needs to feel useful with some degree of the integrity and self-esteem our society places on independence. This book is not a scientific or a theoretical production, but rather, it is an effort to present a compilation of material based upon many real-life experiences with disabled and handicapped people in the development of art and craft therapy at its simplest level. This book differs from other art and craft books in that the ideas presented are not only intended to hold the interest of children and adults but also to meet the needs of professionals and volunteers alike. The explicit instructions with detailed patterns and diagrams are again included due to a favorable response since the first publication in 1977. A section of helpful hints has been added to this edition to serve as a supplementary tool for the project coordinator.

The skills necessary for the artworks in this book are simple enough for the very disabled and handicapped yet not belittling to geriatric patients. Although the projects we suggest are suitable for many ages, we are mainly concerned with daycare and residential programs. Projects were tested with patients ranging from the physically able but very senile to the extremely disabled but mentally alert. The activities are appropriate for those with mental or emotional disability and even enable individuals with physical impairments to use common tools and materials in an essential type of therapeutic recreation.

We hope that the projects described herein will suggest new means of coping with the many idle hours that beset the extremely disabled and handicapped, whether their problems are physical, social, or emotional.

J.G. Cohen
M.C. Wannamaker

ACKNOWLEDGMENTS

It is a pleasure to acknowledge the many friends who have offered their help and have been so gracious as to share their ideas and enthusiasm.

Our wholehearted thanks to B. R. Beaver, Jennifer Kay, and Dr. T. D. Davis!

A special note of appreciation to our family members, who have given us their full support.

And most of all, we thank the residents of Guardian Foundation, Alzheimer's Day Services, Inc., and Nursecare, a group of people who share a wisdom and understanding of life known only to the disabled and handicapped among us.

J.G.C.
M.C.W.

CONTENTS

EXPRESSIVE ARTS FOR THE
VERY DISABLED AND HANDICAPPED
FOR ALL AGES

Chapter One

THE DISABLED
AND HANDICAPPED

Major technological and medical advances are helping to save lives today of those who not long ago would have died. Acknowledging that scientific discovery can never lead to the prevention or cure of all disease and illness, fulfilling activities must be developed for the lives saved by today's degree of technology.

Today there is improved health care available to the poor and those in outlying areas. The premature infant mortality rate is declining along with the birth rate. Research is bringing cancer, heart, and vascular diseases under more control. The net result is a growth in not only the sixty-five-and-over age group but also the number of the enfeebled aged who once would have died. Likewise, premature infants, children, and adults ill with acute infections or the injuries of accidents also live. But they live with gross alterations in physique and with severe impairments in physiological functioning.

Although medicine has made phenomenal advancements, such as those against polio and against blindness caused by an untreated mother's syphilis, realistically, there is little hope that disability and illness will disappear. While effective treatments are being developed for catastrophic illnesses, many diseases such as AIDS, arthritis, Alzheimer's, and paralysis continue to challenge our technological resources. Increasing numbers of babies are born with birth defects due to parental substance abuse and inadequate prenatal care. Illness and disability are not disappearing; rather, the number of extremely disabled people throughout the world is escalating.

Thus it appears that physical disability is often the price of saving lives. In the past, a distinction was made between the terms physically disabled and handicapped. The term disability denoted a medical-physical defect or impairment. Intrinsically, disability referred to an inability to meet certain standards of physical efficiency. In fact, even today disability refers to an inability to meet certain standards of physical efficiency. It differs from disease in that it does not refer to the fundamental biological needs of life. Physical disability might be considered to be the antithesis of capability or physical fitness, while that of illness is health.

Likewise in the past, the term handicapped was a colloquialism for the crippled or physically unfit as well as an impairment in a particular kind of social or psychological behavior. Inherent in this distinction was the fact that handicaps did not always coincide with disabilities. It might be useful to look at an example: Macular Degeneration is an illness: blindness resulting from this illness is a disability; the problem of adjustment in coping with the blindness is a handicap. Thus, it became useful to distinguish between physical limitations and the resultant psychological and social impairments for understanding why people with the same physical disabilities sometimes behaved differently.

Today, many people with physical impairments prefer to be called "disabled" because they feel "handicapped" connotes condescension. However, governmental agencies still use the term "handicapped," and the Council for Exceptional Children publishes articles that use the term "handicapped" in their titles. Thus, the authors of this book use the terms interchangeably with no intent of insensitivity toward the issues involved.

It should be noted that physical disabilities are relative to the culture in which they occur. For example, in our society, a bilateral hand amputee would be disabled. However, in China's traditional culture, when a man was approaching the pinnacle of success, he closed his hands into fists and allowed his fingernails to grow through the palms to the other side. Although he lost the use of his hands, he gained recognition and prestige by showing he had servants to care for him and did not have to resort to common labor. In light of this, it can be said that a disability exists only when a person lacks the means for behavior that his culture deems important.

Although one might attempt to define disability, all delineations are complicated by social judgements. Social prejudice can and does effect behavior. Although serious attempts are made to understand disabilities and handicaps, there is still derisive contempt for the physically and mentally impaired. It is simply a fact that although some physical disabilities are socially handicapping only, they are still perceived by the majority as undesirable. Examples of these social prejudices are those based on physical attributes such as race, gender, and age. Fair or not, these social stereotypes determine how people are expected to behave and what they will be permitted to do. Thus, socially imposed handicaps on people with atypical physiques are important to the overall understanding of physical disability. People raised to think of themselves as "cripples" (a term with so many negative connotations) will behave as they think society expects. An elderly person may respond negatively when hearing such colloquialisms as "over the hill" and "out to pasture."

It is understandable that physical defects and social handicaps place individuals under particular stress. However, except in cases which are almost totally disabling, the significance of these impairments in the development of emotional handicaps depends primarily upon the way the individual evaluates and adjusts to unusual or changed life situations. In many cases, the physical disability is an excuse for, and not the cause of, psychological maladjustment.

The main problems which occur are resignation and feelings of inferiority, self-pity, fear, and hostility. In effect, the individuals listen to society and devaluate themselves accordingly. It is important to note again that the attitude toward the disability seems to be the salient variable in emotional adjustment. Consequently, there is the potential for good adjustment with a severe physical disability and widespread emotional handicaps with only slight physical defects.

Although disability, social handicap, and emotional handicap have been explained independently and separately from each other, combinations of handicaps are the rule rather than the exception. Of course, impairments may be small. However, they are often chronic. Too often, chronically ill patients become isolated and ignored. Few want to spend time with them when they are depressing and exhausting, and their problems are irreversible. A chain reaction occurs. The lessened social interaction of disabled people leads to loneliness and isolation, reducing at the same time their resources for coping with problems. The ensuing stress in turn contributes to illness. The patients begin to play a role of being sick. Is there a better cure for pain or a better balm for emotional ills than feeling useful or playing a truly meaningful role in society? But who will help a grossly impaired person with multiple disabilities and handicaps who lives only because of modern medical miracles at so high a cost?

Chapter Two

EXPRESSIVE ARTS AND CRAFTS

The disabled frequently live in convalescent and nursing homes, away from relatives and friends; strangers are their caretakers. The extremely disabled and handicapped person is left with nothing to do, nothing to talk about, nothing to think about, and nothing for which to live.

Many of the disabled and handicapped cannot truly hope to be returned to society yet need meaningful projects as diversionary activities to give the patients some interest outside themselves and some goals to pursue that are within their ability to function. We have observed an increase in morale among groups of patients who planned and produced projects for use in social service agencies, fundraising activities, and performances for families and friends. So it is that the object of rehabilitation for these long-term patients with no chance of recovery is motivation in terms of socialization and activities resulting in an enhanced sense of self-worth. The projects in this book are designed for such activity.

One of the worst problems faced by the professional or volunteer is the task of motivating the patients. Perhaps when patients experience individual creative success, they may eventually pursue the traditional creative arts that allow self-expression. The importance of expressive arts and crafts activities used in a therapeutic role to enhance feelings of self-worth cannot be stressed enough.

While children can benefit from almost any art or craft idea, some projects may not be appropriate for adults. Even the most enfeebled geriatric patients have a lifetime of experience that tells them right away when some project is simple busy work. On the other hand, meaningful activity is associated with a satisfactory level of self-esteem, positive feelings about life, and higher morale. Success in purposeful projects helps patients fight anxiety caused by loss of identity in an institutionalized setting. With good results on the simple projects presented in the following chapters, these patients will be ready to advance as their self-confidence builds.

Chapter Three

FORMAT AND APPLICATIONS

The projects in this book are rated as to level of difficulty. One asterisk denotes an extremely simple and unchallenging project; two asterisks mark a more difficult project, and so on up to five. (Projects are usually marked with two groups of asterisks to show the range of difficulty.) This is a subjective value judgement on the part of the authors. Just as two people with the same physical disability can have radically different behavior, they also may perform tasks at different levels depending on their interests and motivations.

A project with one asterisk might be very repetitive and excellent therapy for a senile patient, or it might be simple enough for a blind patient. Although a project such as Paper Flowers is suitable for the senile and blind, it might also appeal to more able or alert patients for a shorter period of time.

Each of the projects that has five asterisks necessitates a higher level of eye-hand coordination or more attention to detail. However, when the therapist works bedside in a one-to-one relationship, even the very enfeebled can accomplish most of the projects in this book.

Actually, the rating system is relative at best, as all the projects were designed for an exceptionally low level of ability. It is simply that some projects are better for some impairments, while other projects are better for others. For example, the bold outlines of the patterns for Coasters make them easy to see for the visually impaired, and since any coloring out of lines is cut away from the pattern, it is a good project for hands that shake. Likewise, since tremor often improves or disappears with purposeful function, Potato Print Cards are especially good for patients with Parkinson's disease. On the other hand, paints are not good for shaking hands unless you have very understanding assistants, who do not mind doing extra clean-up duties. If the instructions are read like recipes, the best combinations of disorders and projects will soon be learned.

The activities presented in this book can almost all be completed in one session of approximately one hour. The therapist should be patient, as the participants have nothing but time. Help and interference on a project may produce more finished products per hour but will not help the patients feel a sense of accomplishment. While all patients should be encouraged to participate, they should not be forced. Observation alone is valuable and may eventually lead to participation at another time. Even if patients are passive participants, they enter into the resocialization process. They move toward some degree of independent action within the framework of the social structure of life in their institution.

Although the craft projects in this book are limited to a low level of difficulty, they are truly useful to the patients and others. The projects are separated by chapter as to their particular applications. Some of the uses are multiple, but all in all, the intent of the book is to provide a year's projects (if taken weekly). Some of the activities are more suitable for a holiday while others, such as Strawberries, are good seasonal projects.

The section titled PROJECTS JUST TO ENJOY are meant for the patients themselves. Patients may not want to part with their creations. At the very least, the first or best one of a particular project is usually carried back to the patient's room, and who does not derive pleasure from his own accomplishments?

Keep in mind that not all residents are ambulatory. The section titled PROJECTS FOR USE BY OTHER PATIENTS will offer ambulatory patients opportunities to help others even less fortunate than themselves.

Families play a large role in the lives of patients. They are a link to the outside world. Children want to show their accomplishments for approval. Parents and grandparents want some token to give visitors, as they often do not have the means to shop for gifts. The PROJECTS TO GIVE TO FAMILY MEMBERS are designed for this purpose.

Patients often produce item after item for family members who never come to visit. The greatest sense of self-esteem for these patients seems to come from PROJECTS FOR USE BY AGENCIES. Most cities have volunteer bureaus which are hungry for any type of handicraft. They will distribute the projects to appropriate recipients and will send a nice letter of appreciation to show the patients. The Veterans Administration, children's hospitals, schools, and church bazaars are only a few of the organizations that will make good use of the projects. Police and fire departments may be asked what they can use. Bookmarks can be given to libraries. All projects should be given with a note about how and why they were made. There should be no embarrassment about the quality of workmanship or about asking for a letter of appreciation in return for the projects.

PROJECTS TO SELL may be marketed in the institution's boutique or gift shop. For so long, personal worth has been measured by financial success; this idea dies hard. Some patients only feel useful with some degree of the integrity and esteem our society places upon independence when their projects are sold.

Chapter Four

HELPFUL HINTS

In working with the elderly or those patients with mental or physical impairments, remember to take into consideration their decreased ability to learn or retain new information; longer periods of time are needed to accomplish seemingly simple tasks. Additionally, difficulties with fine motor skills require attention to selecting projects that minimize frustration and stress. Incentives are a must; many are taught that work is good and idleness is sinful. Thus, the projects attempted must be deemed valuable. The therapist is not apt to pull the wool over anybody's eyes with simple busy work.

From a therapeutic perspective, the process of participation with the group and involvement in the project itself is more important than the finished product. Sometimes participants will not like or want their projects; the activities director need not insist. Perhaps another patient would like it, or it might be displayed in the activities room (with the patient's permission). Remember to use discretion in giving compliments; honest and helpful criticism is always preferable to insincere flattery.

Ideally, the arts and crafts therapist should be familiar with the physical and mental status of each patient—what each patient can and cannot do. More often than not, impromptu assessments are necessary to determine the patients' willingness and ability to participate in an activity. Plan ahead for different levels of ability within a group. For example, some patterns may be predrawn, while others can draw their own design in projects such as Dresser Scarves. Preassembly of some projects can be helpful for the extremely impaired participants. A good deal of preparation makes for foolproof projects; however, be sure to allow for creativity and self-expression, which may evolve after successful experiences with patterns. Completed samples of each project are effective aides to instruction and motivation.

The preparation done at home for the teaching of expressive arts and crafts is often grueling. But if the therapist pulls threads and draws patterns on dresser scarves while patients watch, and if the patients are then told to color them, they will feel that they are not doing much. But if patients come into a room and the scarves are ready to color, they will not think too much about how the scarves got there. The project becomes theirs. Any preparation ahead of time is well worth the effort.

11

There are as many personalities as there are people (and sometimes more!); therefore, it would be best for a therapist to know individual traits and abilities. Unfortunately, the therapist is often only a part-time activities director or volunteer. What should a therapist do when faced with a shortage of volunteers and twenty-five apprehensive, enfeebled patients waiting to feel useful to themselves and society? The therapist can hardly tat with one and oil paint with another, throw clay pots and do woodwork, needlepoint, and macrame. Projects with general appeal and a low level of difficulty are needed. The problem is that simple projects are often looked upon as child's play by adults and, to quote an elderly patient whose therapist helped with a detailed project, "You do it for us and then tell us how good we are—nonsense!"

Supplies, of course, should be safe and nontoxic. Senile patients often put almost anything into their mouths. Sharp scissors should rarely be used in any group. There are a number of economical ways of acquiring craft supplies, short of stealing. Seeds, plastic foam meat trays, produce baskets, cans, medicine cups, etc., are readily available and were intentionally chosen as materials for the projects in this book. Be sure to ask the kitchen staff to save these items for you. The Yellow Pages will list manufacturers and distributors of boxes, fabric, buttons, trim, cans, colored paper, etc. You will often find these companies generous in their donations of materials. Nature may be used as a veritable storehouse of supplies; collection of nature materials offers an opportunity for a group activity, where applicable.

Name tags are helpful to both the patient and therapist. Using the patient's name frequently affirms recognition and builds self-esteem.

Rapport and trust between the patient and therapist are essential in order to gain cooperation. This, more than anything else, often tests the therapist's or volunteer's ability to present a successful program of activities. In meeting the disabled, it may be difficult to get past the handicap stigma. Nonverbal behavior gives one away. If one is constrained, nervous, or stilted, the patients will be embarrassed. Handicapped people can learn to cope with their affliction in time, but the embarrassment the impairment causes others is almost unbearable to the disabled. The best advice that can be given is to "be honest and be yourself." The patients know their situation; the therapist knows their situation. Reality must not be denied, and yet one must continue in spite of it. Illness is a part of the full circle of life, as is death. Research today points to the need for honesty with all people, even the terminally ill. Since reality is hard enough to cope with, the patient should not be asked to deal with make-believe too. Help should not be given unless asked for; speak directly to the individual in a normal tone. Deafness is not synonymous with paraplegia.

The infirm can be fun and interesting to talk to, and they are very grateful for anything that is done for them. They seem to have a wisdom and understanding of life that would be well worthwhile to learn. Of course, some patients are moody at times or difficult to help. Some are withdrawn and often try the therapist's patience in attempting to motivate them. The therapist should try to realize they are ill and infirm. While the therapist helps the patient do something useful and feel worthwhile, the patient will be helping the therapist do something useful and feel worthwhile. It is only a value judgement to say who does the best job!

Chapter Five

CRAFT PROJECTS JUST TO ENJOY

HIDDEN TREASURES

Level of difficulty: *****

MATERIALS: A portable microphone, overhead projector, instruction sheets, and materials appropriate to the project selected, corsage or boutonniere for the honored speaker or performer.

APPLICATIONS: Many people enjoy sharing their special interests and skills. Group interaction is facilitated by this activity.

PREPARATION BEFORE CRAFT SESSION: You may have access to case histories that mention special interests or hobbies. If not, try group or individual "treasure hunts," learning about each others' special talents. You may also want to contact family members, who may have kept musical instruments, recordings, photographs, paintings, quilts, etc. From this information, you will be able to determine the supplies and arrangements necessary for the program you will develop.

Your community may offer a wealth of professionals and skilled amateurs who would be willing to lead a program.

CRAFT SESSION: Introduce participants in the program. Present the corsage or boutonniere with thanks to the speaker or performer. If necessary, utilize a portable microphone to amplify weak voices and accommodate the hearing impaired. Either have the honored speakers/performers share special talents or have sessions based upon those particular hobbies or interests.

HIDDEN TREASURES

SHARE SPECIAL TALENTS
SUCH AS QUILTING
OR WOODWORKING

BEADS

Level of difficulty: *-*****

MATERIALS: Salt, flour, vegetable colorings, darning needle, cord such as No. 30 crochet cotton, round toothpicks, wax paper, dried seeds, and old broken strands of beads, nail polish, plastic self-hardening clay (optional).

APPLICATIONS: By varying the colors and shapes, you can make many attractive strings. By varying the lengths of the strings, you can make bracelets, necklaces, or belts. Some people with fairly nimble fingers may want to tie a small knot between each bead or seed to make a more attractive strand.

PREPARATION BEFORE CRAFT SESSION: Mix two-thirds of a cup of salt, a cup of flour, one-third of a cup of water, and two or three drops of vegetable coloring. This will form a heavy dough. Make the dough in a variety of colors. To prepare the seeds for stringing, soak the seeds in water for a day or two. Then pierce a hole with a needle in each seed. You may want to paint some of the seeds with nail polish.

CRAFT SESSION: Have each person roll a small amount of the dough between the palms of his hands to shape it. Make a hole with a toothpick in the center of each bead as soon as it is finished. Lay the beads on wax paper to dry, or the beads can be dried on toothpicks which have been secured in a styrofoam base. This method keeps the round shape of the beads.

STRINGING BEADS

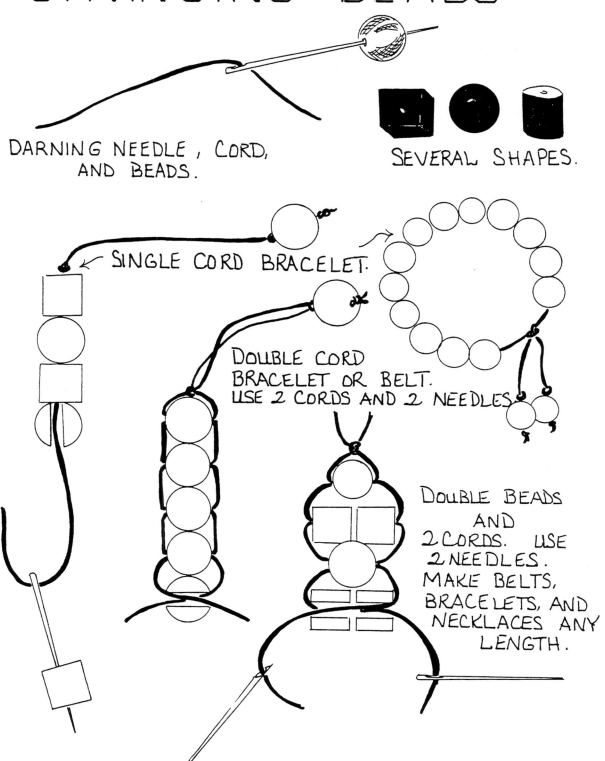

DARNING NEEDLE, CORD, AND BEADS.

SEVERAL SHAPES.

SINGLE CORD BRACELET.

DOUBLE CORD BRACELET OR BELT. USE 2 CORDS AND 2 NEEDLES.

DOUBLE BEADS AND 2 CORDS. USE 2 NEEDLES. MAKE BELTS, BRACELETS, AND NECKLACES ANY LENGTH.

SALT BEADS

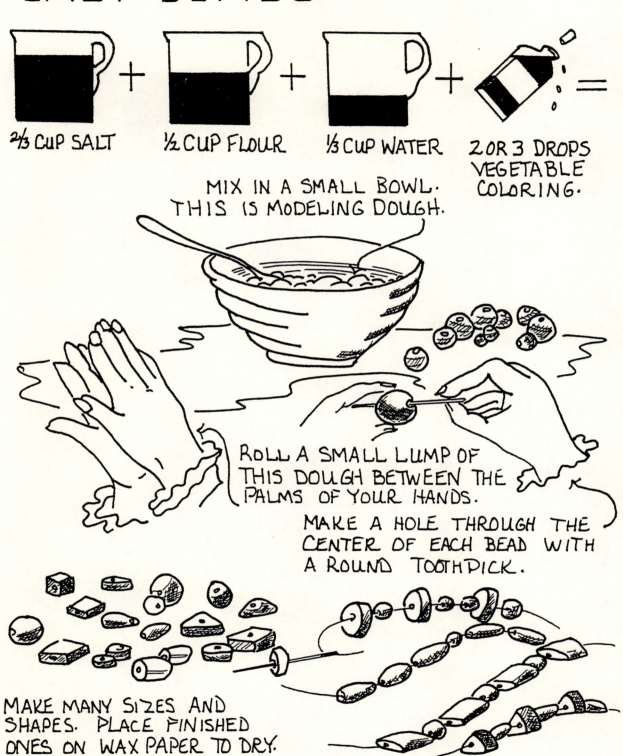

2/3 CUP SALT + 1/2 CUP FLOUR + 1/3 CUP WATER + 2 OR 3 DROPS VEGETABLE COLORING. =

MIX IN A SMALL BOWL. THIS IS MODELING DOUGH.

ROLL A SMALL LUMP OF THIS DOUGH BETWEEN THE PALMS OF YOUR HANDS.

MAKE A HOLE THROUGH THE CENTER OF EACH BEAD WITH A ROUND TOOTHPICK.

MAKE MANY SIZES AND SHAPES. PLACE FINISHED ONES ON WAX PAPER TO DRY.

SEED BEADS

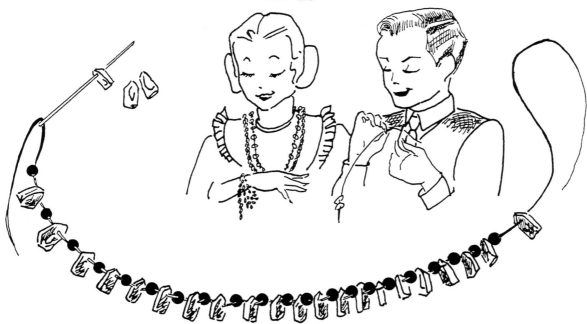

STRING SEEDS AND BEADS OF OLD
BROKEN STRANDS.

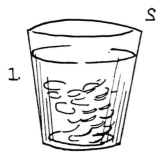

1.

SOAK THE SEEDS
IN WATER FOR A
DAY OR TWO.

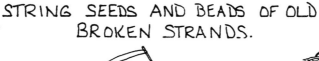

2.

PIERCE A HOLE WITH
A NEEDLE, THEN STRING.

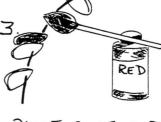

3.

RED

PAINT SOME OF THE
SEEDS WITH NAIL
POLISH.

USE — BEANS- WATERMELON SEEDS -CANTELOPE SEEDS-
CORN -PUMPKIN SEEDS- SQUASH SEEDS-
SUNFLOWER SEEDS.

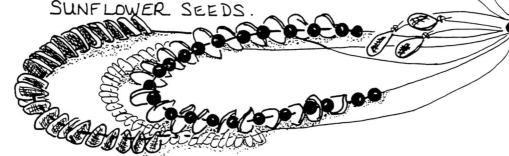

MOSAIC

Level of difficulty: *-*****

MATERIALS: Wallpaper (samples are fine), dozens of buttons, craft glue, brush; any other interesting objects such as loose beads, pearls, seeds, plastic produce baskets (all optional).

APPLICATIONS: These intricate mosaics are pleasant to view when hung on the wall opposite a bed, or place small ones on little easels on dressers or night stands.

PREPARATION BEFORE CRAFT SESSION: None.

CRAFT SESSION: Let each person choose a piece of wallpaper that especially appeals to him. Brush the paper with glue, a section at a time. Then applique the paper with buttons. Add other objects if desired. Plastic produce baskets can be cut into rectangles. They will look like stained glass windows when glued over wallpaper that has a small design on it.

MOSAIC

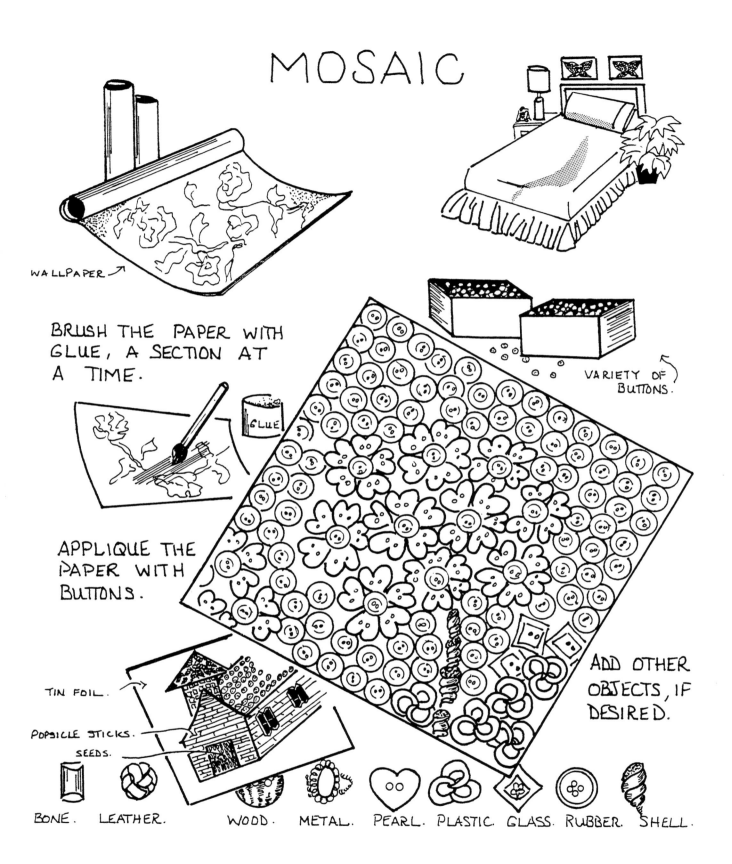

WALLPAPER

BRUSH THE PAPER WITH GLUE, A SECTION AT A TIME.

GLUE

APPLIQUE THE PAPER WITH BUTTONS.

VARIETY OF BUTTONS.

TIN FOIL.

POPSICLE STICKS.

SEEDS.

ADD OTHER OBJECTS, IF DESIRED.

BONE.   LEATHER.   WOOD.   METAL.   PEARL.   PLASTIC.   GLASS.   RUBBER.   SHELL.

CACTUS TERRARIUMS

Level of difficulty: *-*****

MATERIALS: Wire clothes hangers, and wire cutter, or wooden skewer, empty glass jars, plastic spoons, potting soil, sand in a variety of colors, one cactus for each terrarium, wet towels.

APPLICATIONS: A terrarium is a small garden in a glass. These colorful terrariums can decorate a window sill or night stand and do not require regular watering by forgetful minds.

PREPARATION BEFORE CRAFT SESSION: Cut the hangers into 10-inch lengths. Divide the sands and soil into several containers so that each person has a nice selection with which to work.

CRAFT SESSION: Let each person fill a jar with layers of colored sand until it is about two-thirds full. Then using a wire hanger stick, or wooden skewer, glide the wire down the inside of the jar until it touches the bottom and lift it back along its original path. Repeat this procedure all the way around the jar to create an interesting design in the sand. Be careful not to shake the jars, or the colored sands will mix. When the design is complete, add a layer of potting soil and plant a cactus. Clean messy hands with wet towels.

CACTUS TERRARIUMS

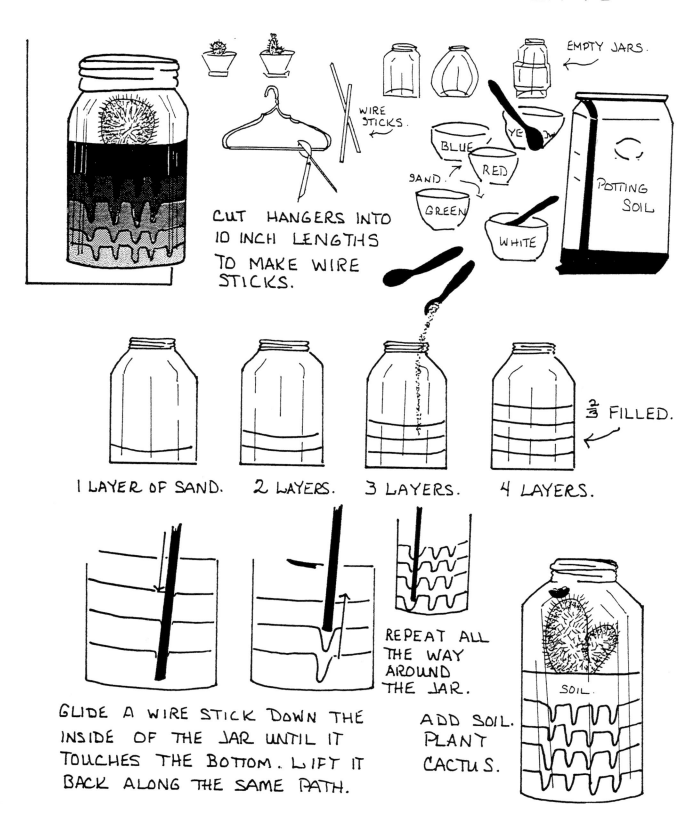

CUT HANGERS INTO 10 INCH LENGTHS TO MAKE WIRE STICKS.

WIRE STICKS.

EMPTY JARS.

BLUE

YELLOW

RED

SAND.

GREEN

WHITE

POTTING SOIL

1 LAYER OF SAND.   2 LAYERS.   3 LAYERS.   4 LAYERS.

2/3 FILLED.

GLIDE A WIRE STICK DOWN THE INSIDE OF THE JAR UNTIL IT TOUCHES THE BOTTOM. LIFT IT BACK ALONG THE SAME PATH.

REPEAT ALL THE WAY AROUND THE JAR.

ADD SOIL. PLANT CACTUS.

SOIL.

WOODEN HORSE

Level of difficulty: **-*****

MATERIALS: Fabric scraps, craft glue, scissors, spring clothespins, green yarn, wood stain, varnish, brushes, sandpaper, wood scraps, hammer, nails, jigsaw.

APPLICATIONS: Although the preparation before the craft session is somewhat tedious, the craft session itself is a lot of fun. The finished horses make an appealing toy for children or an eye-catching note or photo holder for adults. The Nursecare Nursing Center (of Charlotte, North Carolina) combined a western music day with the craft session. Patients kept their horses as souvenirs of a happy occasion. Before the horses were attached to their bases, some of the men sanded the wood. Often men are thrilled to do this type of work even when they do not care to participate in an actual craft session.

PREPARATION BEFORE CRAFT SESSION: Using a jigsaw, cut out horses and bases. Sand the wood. Then stain and varnish the bases, horses, and clothespins (one for each horse). Patterns can be enlarged to any size. Attach the horses to the bases with nails and glue.

CRAFT SESSION: Using fabric scraps, cut out a mane, tail, saddle, feet and covering for the base. Using green yarn, cut out lots of grass. Glue the cloth to the horse. It is easiest to apply glue with a brush onto the horse and then lay the fabric on top of the glue. Sprinkle grass around the feet and attach the clothespin head.

WOODEN HORSE

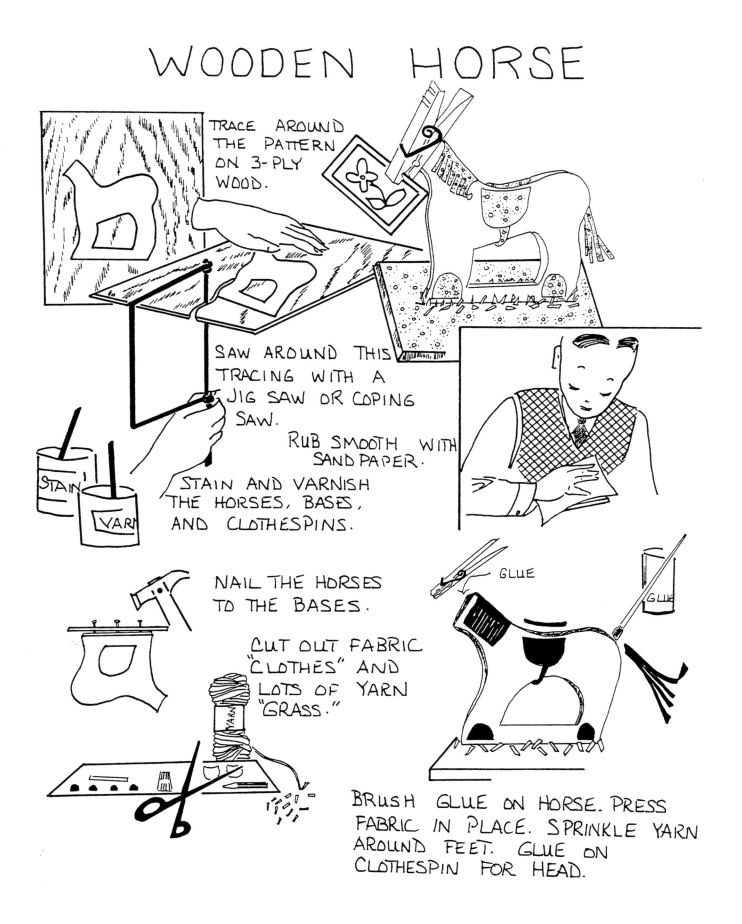

TRACE AROUND THE PATTERN ON 3-PLY WOOD.

SAW AROUND THIS TRACING WITH A JIG SAW OR COPING SAW.

RUB SMOOTH WITH SAND PAPER.

STAIN AND VARNISH THE HORSES, BASES, AND CLOTHESPINS.

NAIL THE HORSES TO THE BASES.

CUT OUT FABRIC "CLOTHES" AND LOTS OF YARN "GRASS."

BRUSH GLUE ON HORSE. PRESS FABRIC IN PLACE. SPRINKLE YARN AROUND FEET. GLUE ON CLOTHESPIN FOR HEAD.

STAIN

VARN

YARN

GLUE

GLUE

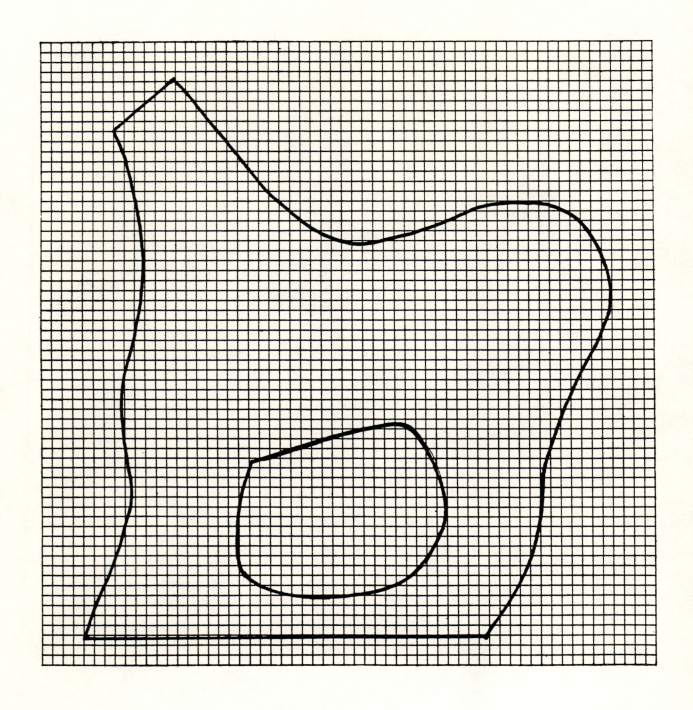

PATTERN FOR WOODEN HORSE

PATTERNS FOR WOODEN HORSE

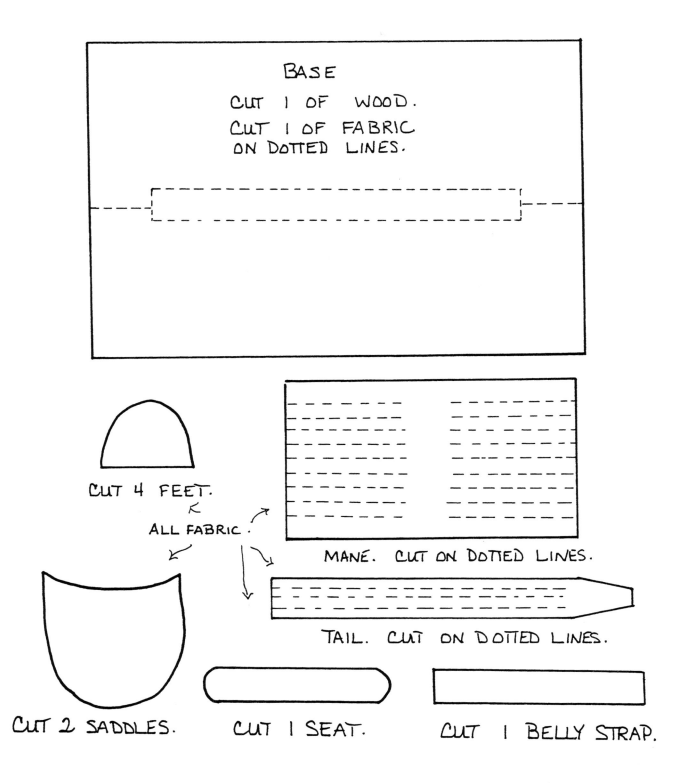

BASE

CUT 1 OF WOOD.

CUT 1 OF FABRIC ON DOTTED LINES.

CUT 4 FEET.

ALL FABRIC.

MANE. CUT ON DOTTED LINES.

TAIL. CUT ON DOTTED LINES.

CUT 2 SADDLES.

CUT 1 SEAT.

CUT 1 BELLY STRAP.

MATCHING FABRIC NOTECARDS

Level of difficulty: *-*****

MATERIALS: Two yards, unbleached muslin, felt marking pens in a variety of colors, pinking shears, glue, drawing paper, envelopes, scissors, ball point pen, rubber bands, or string. You may prefer water colors, stamp pads, sponge applications, etc.

APPLICATIONS: These cards become *matched* when the very large piece of decorated cloth is cut into many small pieces. These notecards are always handy for patients to give to special visitors or to write friends on special occasions. The notes can also be used for invitations to special events or fundraisers.

PREPARATION BEFORE CRAFT SESSION: Cut dozens of pieces of drawing paper which, when folded in half, will fit the envelopes you have for the notes. On the bottom of the back of each folded note, print "made by ----------." You may use beige drawing paper to match the muslin, but this is not necessary.

CRAFT SESSION: Using felt pens in a variety of colors, have each person decorate the cloth until it is solidly covered with color. Hit the cloth at random to make dozens of dots or dashes; scribble in large or small circles; draw pictures; sign names; use imagination. The idea is for everyone to contribute to the overall coloring of the fabric. Then cut the material with pinking shears to fit each folded note. Glue the fabric to the note. Stack the notes with an equal set of envelopes. Secure the notes and envelopes with rubber bands or string.

MATCHING FABRIC NOTECARDS

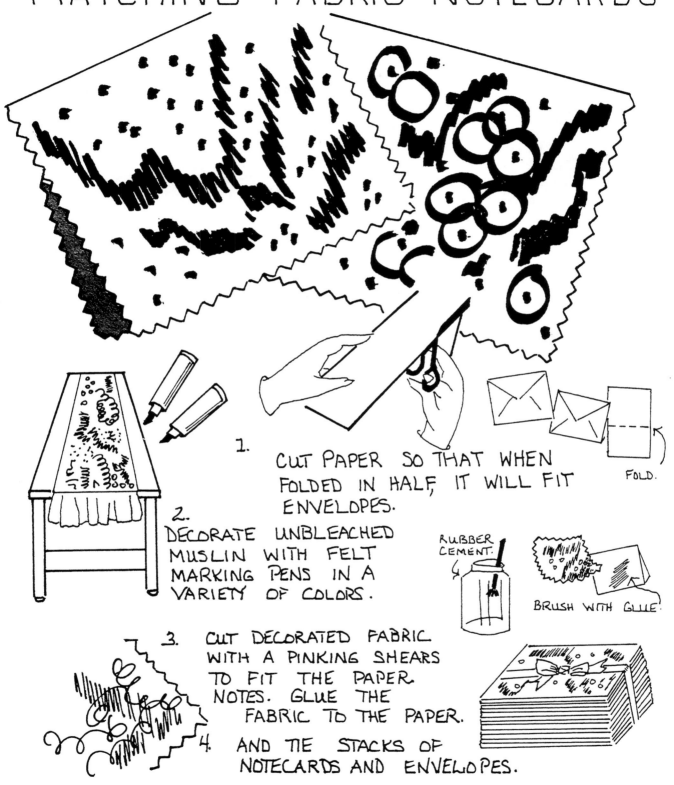

1. CUT PAPER SO THAT WHEN FOLDED IN HALF, IT WILL FIT ENVELOPES.

FOLD.

2. DECORATE UNBLEACHED MUSLIN WITH FELT MARKING PENS IN A VARIETY OF COLORS.

RUBBER CEMENT.

BRUSH WITH GLUE.

3. CUT DECORATED FABRIC WITH A PINKING SHEARS TO FIT THE PAPER NOTES. GLUE THE FABRIC TO THE PAPER.

4. AND TIE STACKS OF NOTECARDS AND ENVELOPES.

DRESSER SCARVES

Level of difficulty: *-*****

MATERIALS: Unbleached muslin (or any inexpensive, pastel unpatterned fabric), scissors, wax crayons, iron, wax paper, masking tape.

APPLICATIONS: The illustration shows you how to make a dresser scarf by applying this method of decoration. After you have learned the method, you can make other decorated textiles such as placemats, dollhouse curtains, or handkerchiefs.

PREPARATION BEFORE CRAFT SESSION: Pull the threads, one at a time, along each edge to make the fringe; or hem the scarves with a blanket stitch. Draw a pattern on the scarves with a pencil. You can enlarge or reduce patterns on a photocopy machine. Coloring books offer other patterns. Then, using the masking tape, tape each doily to the table in front of each person so that it will not slide around.

CRAFT SESSION: Have each person color the entire design with wax crayons, using any colors they wish. Better results are obtained if they color with the weave of the material, namely, across and lengthwise. Be sure to put each person's name on his scarf before untaping it. Then set the crayon yourself by melting it into the cloth so that it does not wash out or wear off. To do this, place piece of wax paper over the crayoned doily. Top the wax paper with a single layer of newspaper to protect the iron. Then press it with a very warm iron. *Be careful* that the people with whom you are working cannot reach the iron or its cord. Note that there are permanent fabric markers available if appropriate for your participants.

DRESSER SCARVES

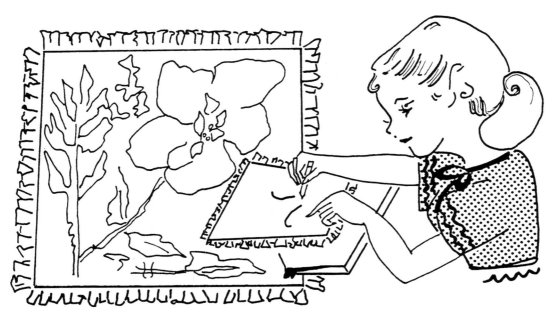

THIS IS A DRESSER SCARF.
IT IS 15 INCHES SQUARE.

1.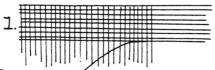

PULL THE THREADS OUT ALONG
THE EDGES TO MAKE THE
FRINGE.

2. TAPE THE SCARF TO THE
TABLE SO IT WON'T SLIDE.

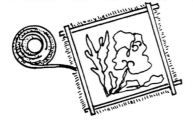

3. DRAW THE DESIGN WITH WAX
CRAYONS.

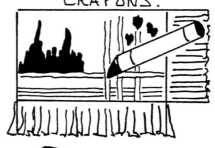

4.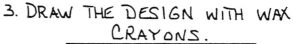

PLACE A PAPER OVER THE SCARF
AND PRESS WITH A VERY WARM IRON.

5. THESE ARE OTHER
IDEAS.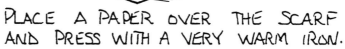

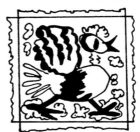

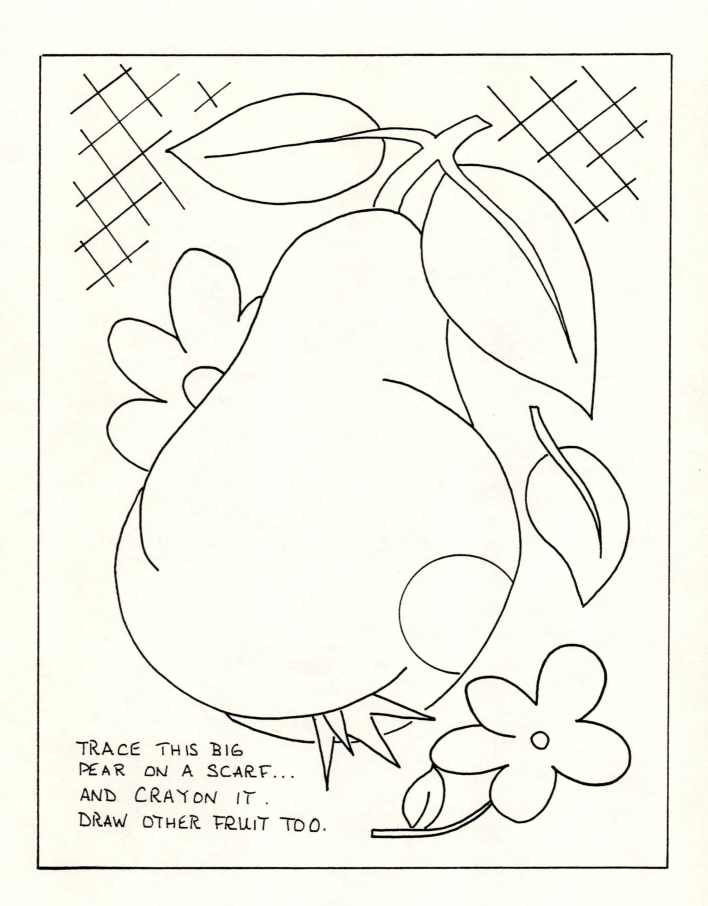

TRACE THIS BIG
PEAR ON A SCARF...
AND CRAYON IT.
DRAW OTHER FRUIT TOO.

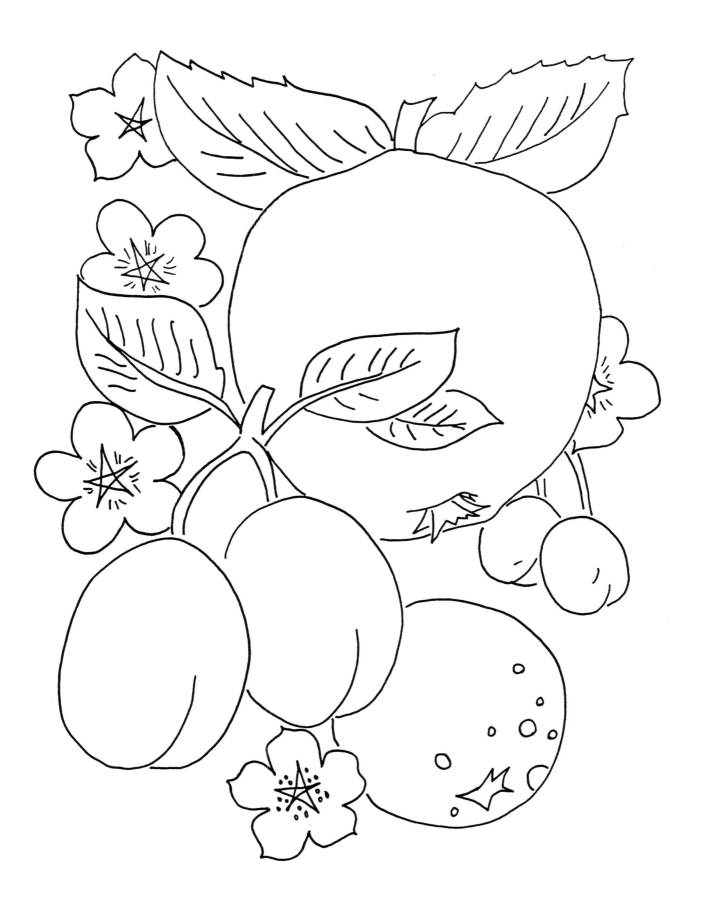

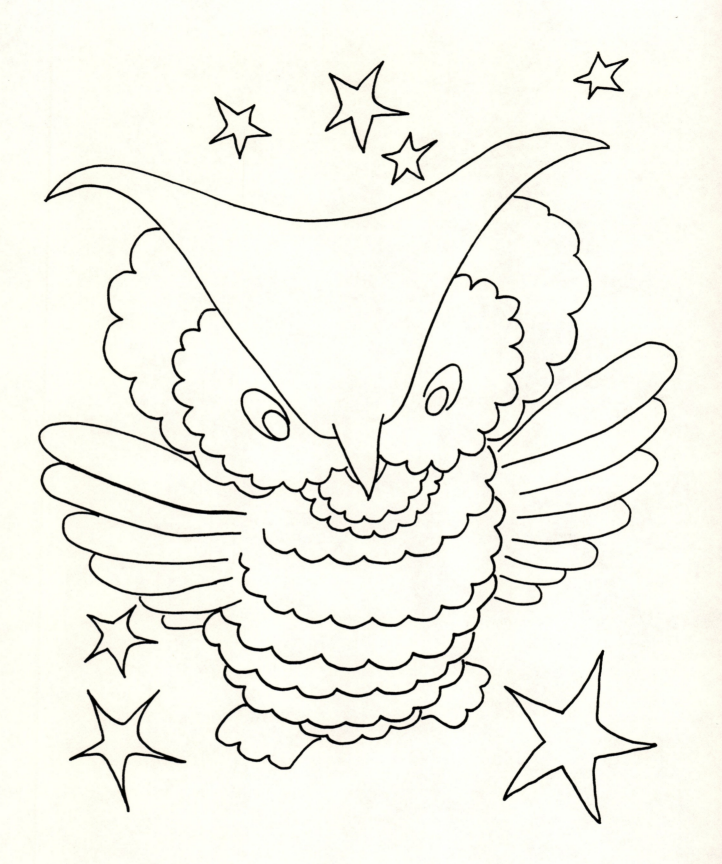

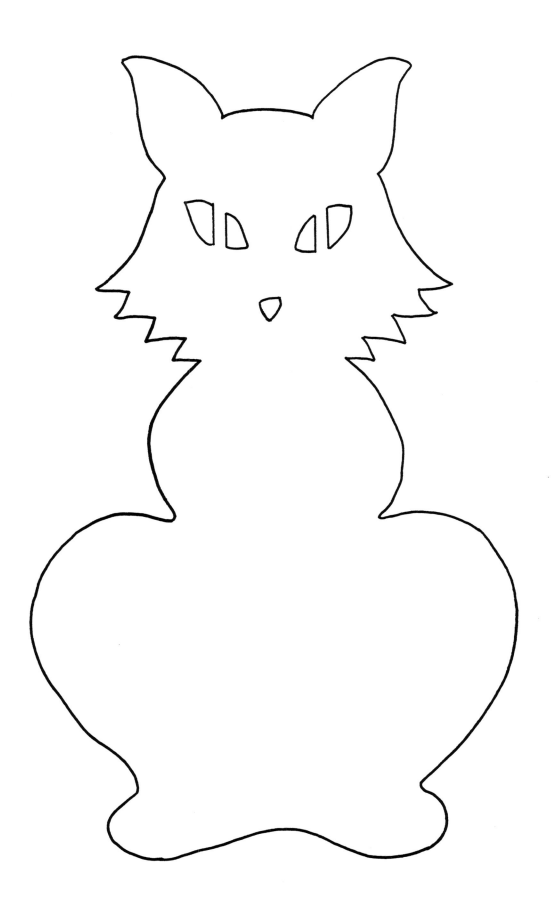

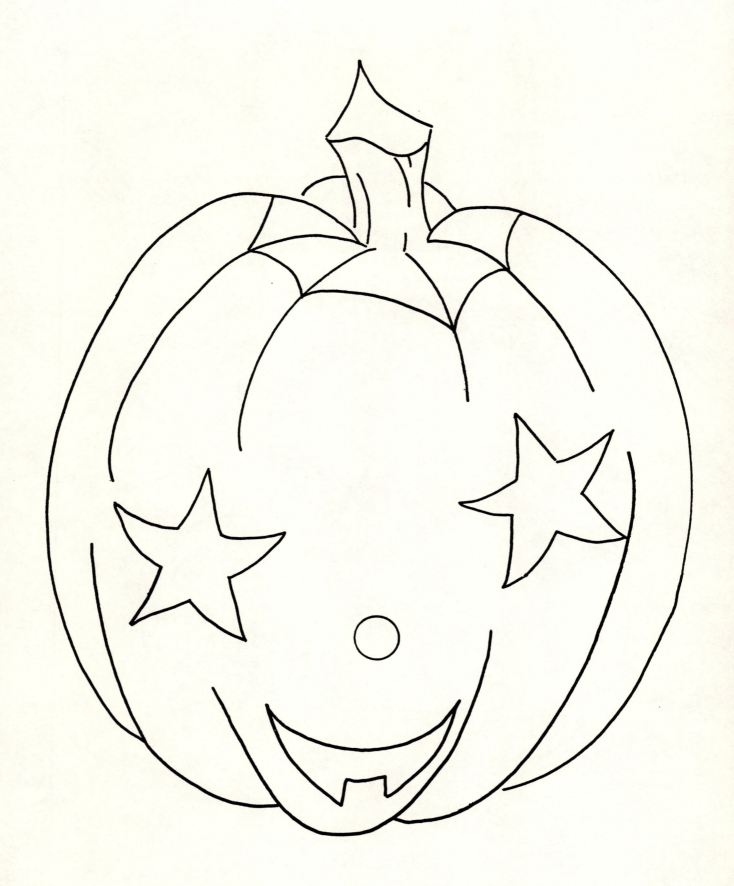

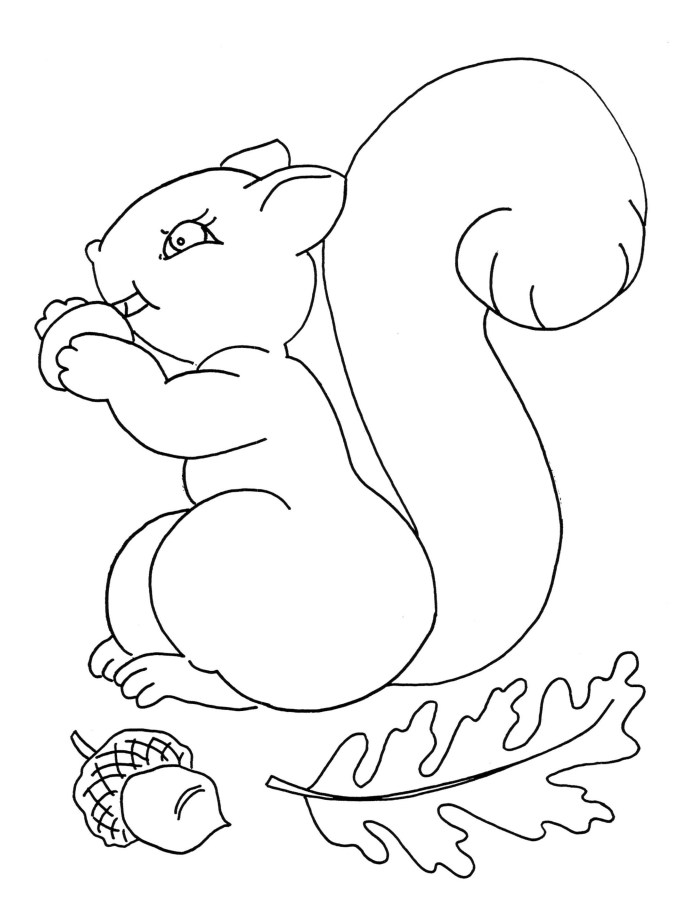

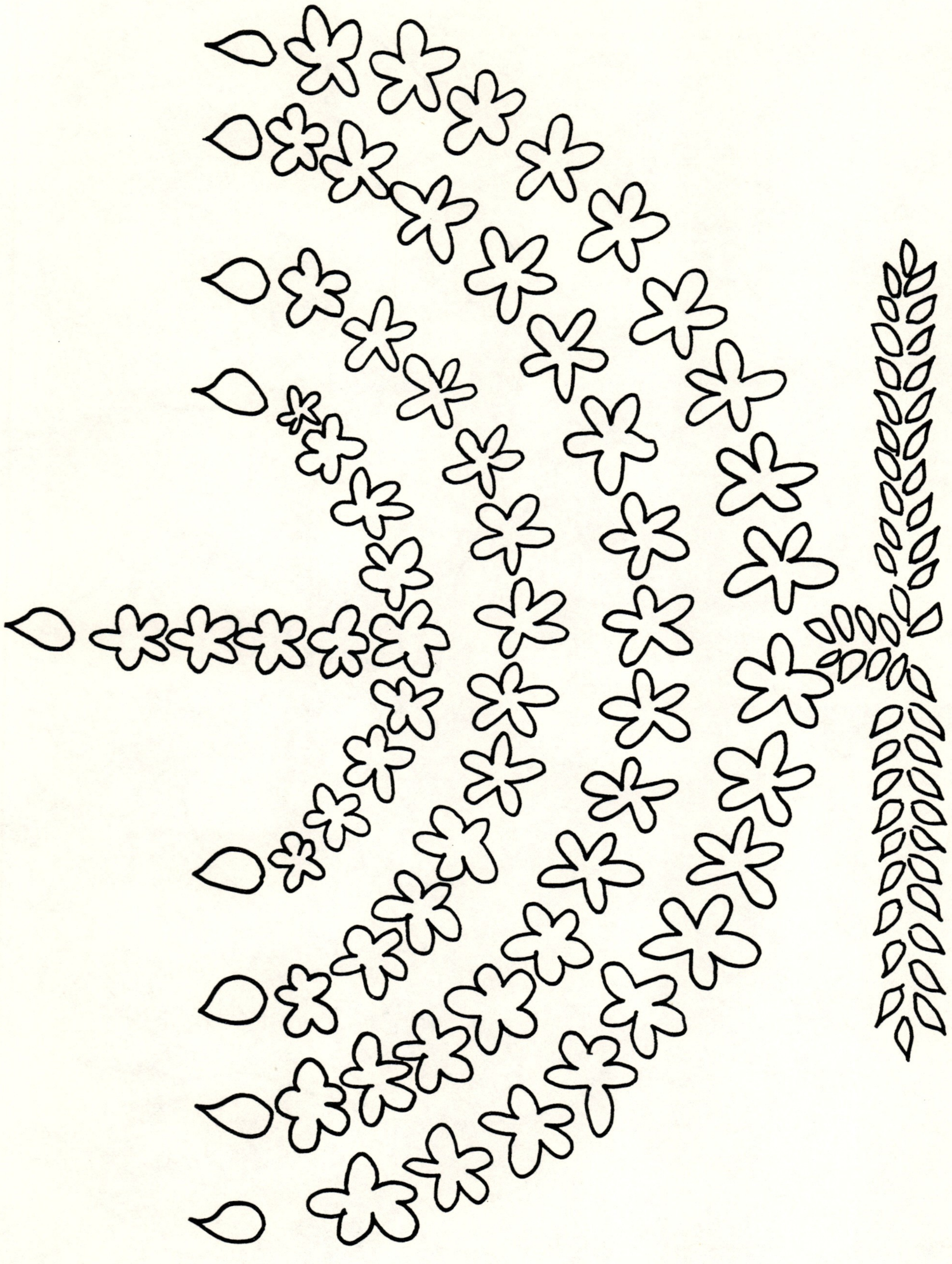

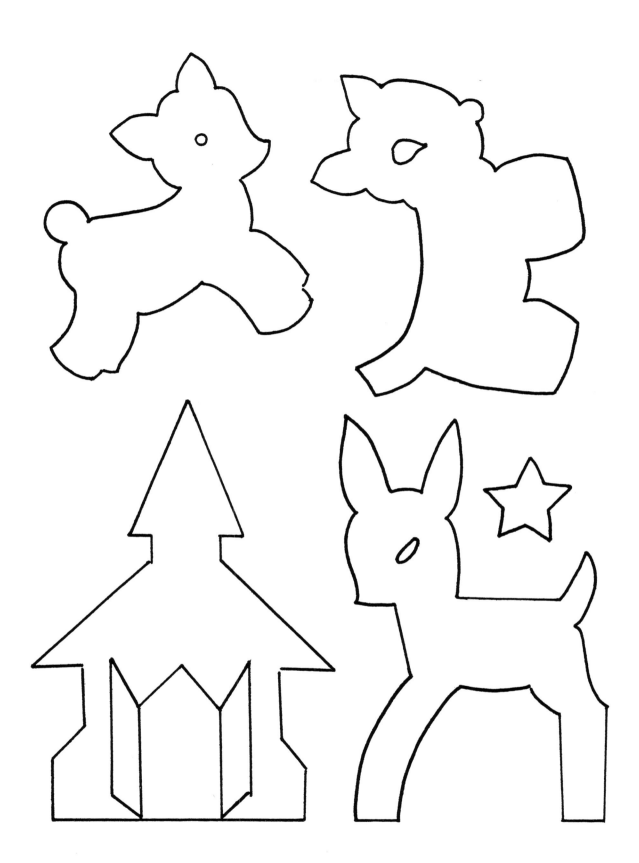

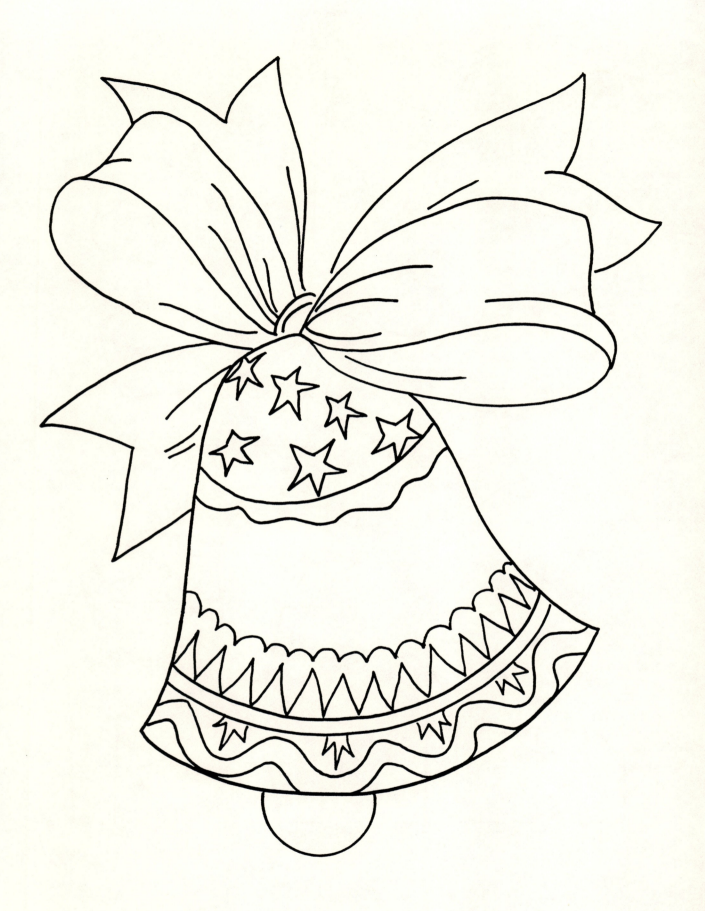

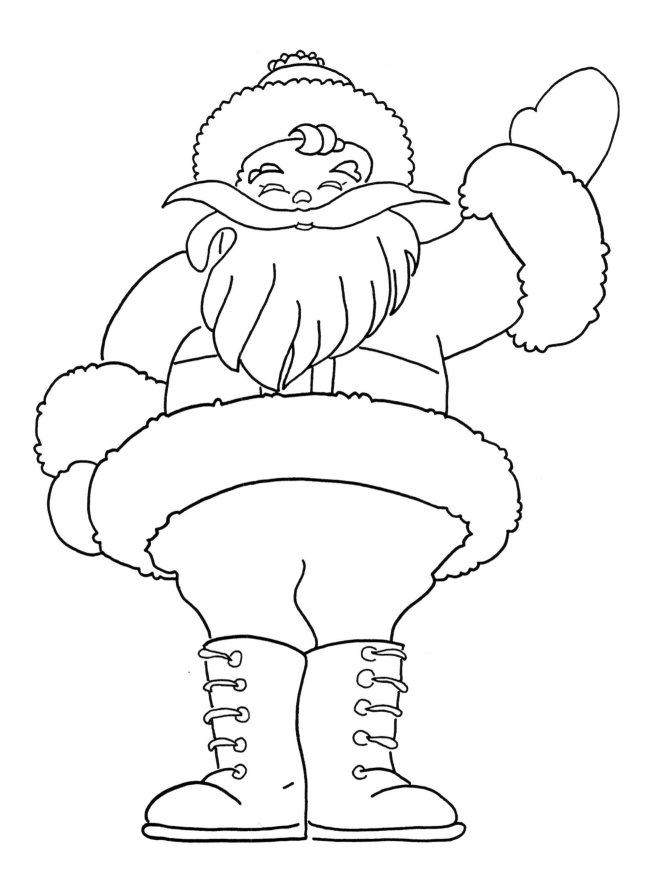

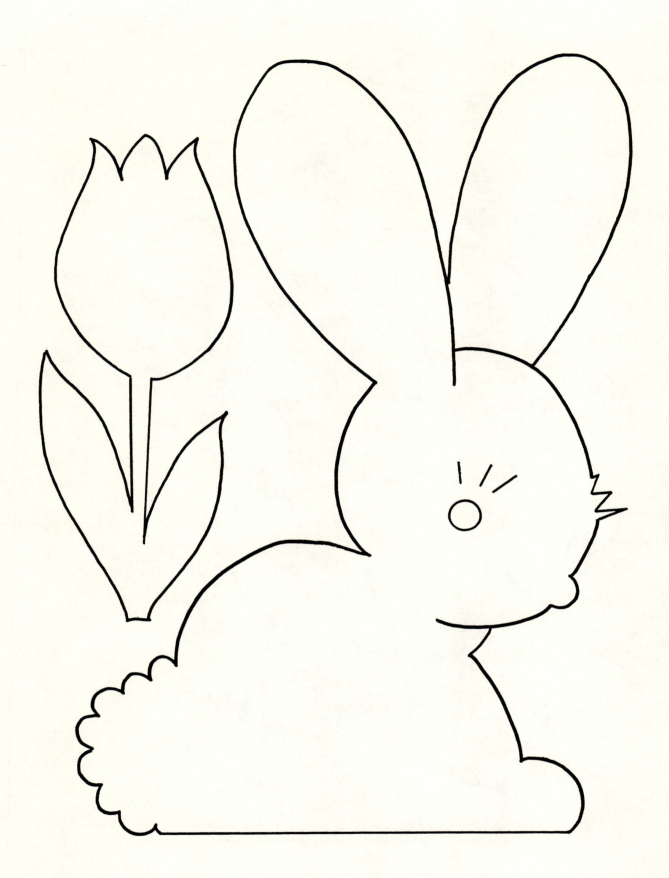

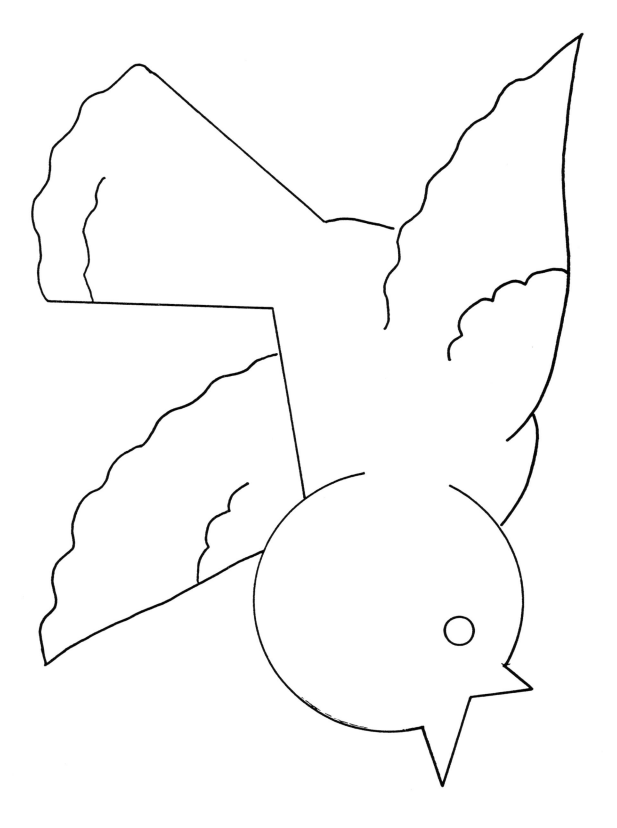

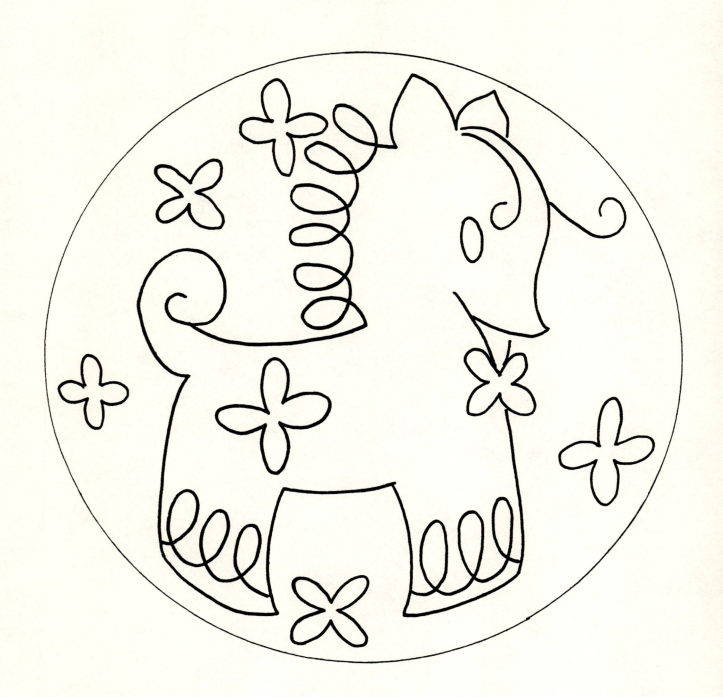

WALL POCKET

Level of difficulty: *-***

MATERIALS: Glue stick, scissors, paper plates, felt marking pens in a variety of colors, paper punch, paper fasteners, pencil, yarn, tacks.

APPLICATIONS: These wall pockets are nice to save special letters or pretty clippings from magazines to use for other projects.

PREPARATION BEFORE CRAFT SESSION: Cut enough plates in half to make one half for each whole plate. Each person should have one whole plate and one half plate. Draw simple designs with a pencil on the back of the half plates. Using glue stick, secure a whole plate (right side up) and half plate (wrong side up) in front of each person.

CRAFT SESSION: Have each person decorate and color the plates using the felt pens. You may substitute tempera paints or crayon. Remove the plates from the table. Hold the half plate onto the whole plate and punch five holes along the edge. Fasten the plates together with paper fasteners through the holes you have punched. Punch two more holes at the top, each about 1½ inches from the center. Tie a piece of yarn through these holes so that the plates can be hung up and used for a wall pocket. See that each person gets a tack and help, if necessary, to hang his pocket.

WALL POCKET

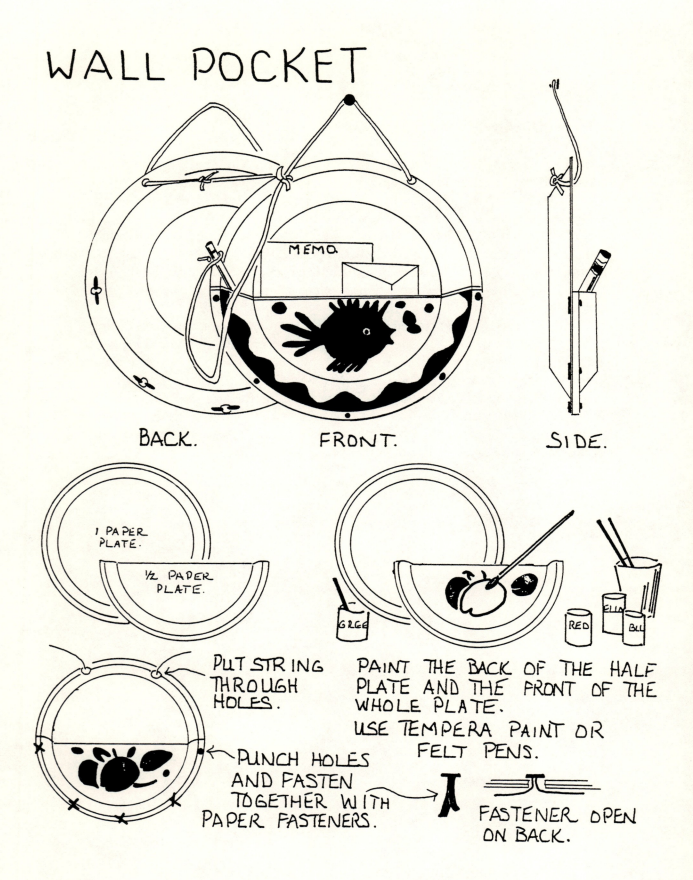

BACK.   FRONT.   SIDE.

1 PAPER PLATE.

½ PAPER PLATE.

GREE

RED ELLA BLU

PUT STRING THROUGH HOLES.

PAINT THE BACK OF THE HALF PLATE AND THE FRONT OF THE WHOLE PLATE.
USE TEMPERA PAINT OR FELT PENS.

PUNCH HOLES AND FASTEN TOGETHER WITH PAPER FASTENERS.

FASTENER OPEN ON BACK.

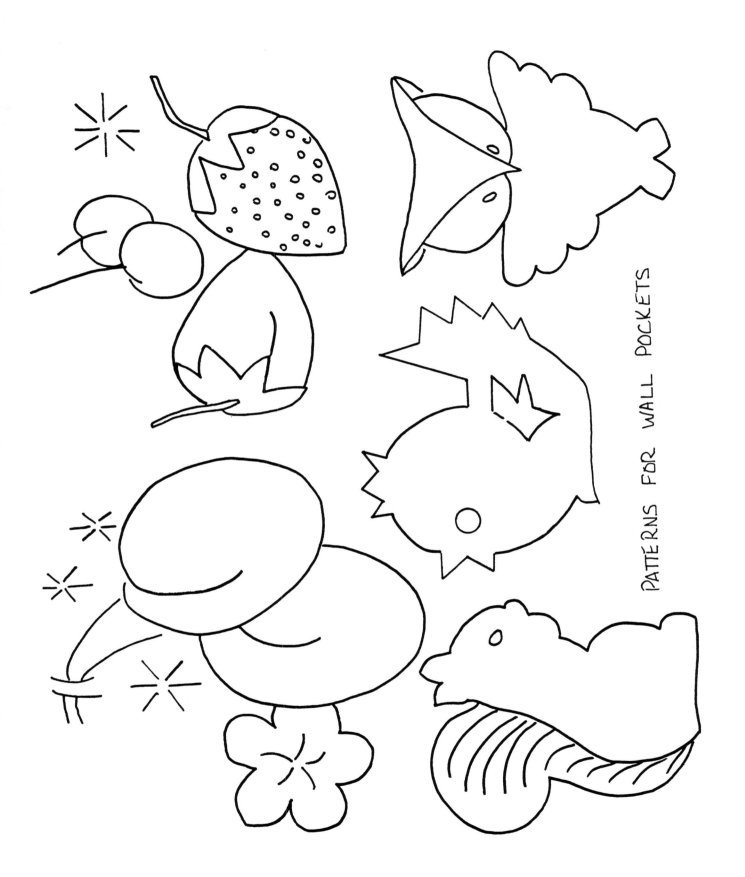

PATTERNS FOR WALL POCKETS

PATCHWORK POTS

Level of difficulty: *-*****

MATERIALS: Clay or plastic flower pots in a variety of sizes, craft glue, brushes, water, empty plastic containers, pinking shears, fabric scraps, ric rac (very narrow, preferably), pen, varnish or craft glaze (optional).

APPLICATIONS: These patchwork pots are absolutely beautiful and foolproof. Gingham or calico squares do not have to be matched to be attractive. However, many older persons enjoy working out intricate designs with the fabric reminiscent of quilting parties in earlier years. Cuttings of rapid growing plants (baby tears and grape ivy) can be planted in the finished pots. Relatives and friends admire the work and often place special orders for pots in particular colors. Favorite combinations are red, yellow, and green or red, white and blue.

Even a partially blind person can paint glue on a pot, and a partner can arrange the fabric squares on the pot. Shaking hands find this to be a confidence building project.

PREPARATION BEFORE CRAFT SESSION: Mix craft glue with a little water until it is the consistency of white glue. Using a pinking shears, cut out dozens of fabric squares approximately 1 inch by 1 inch.

CRAFT SESSION: Put each person's name on the bottom of his pot. This will come in handy when you return the pot with a plant in it. Brush glue on the pot, a section at a time. Arrange the squares attractively on the glue. Be certain to overlap each square slightly so that the pot will not show through the cloth. Then trim the pot with ric rac both vertically around the pot and also around the circumference of the upper and lower rim and bottom of the pot.

After the pot dries, apply several coats of the glue and water mixture over the entire pot, letting it dry between each application. If you like, seal the pot with acrylic based polyurethane. There are no fumes.

PATCHWORK POTS

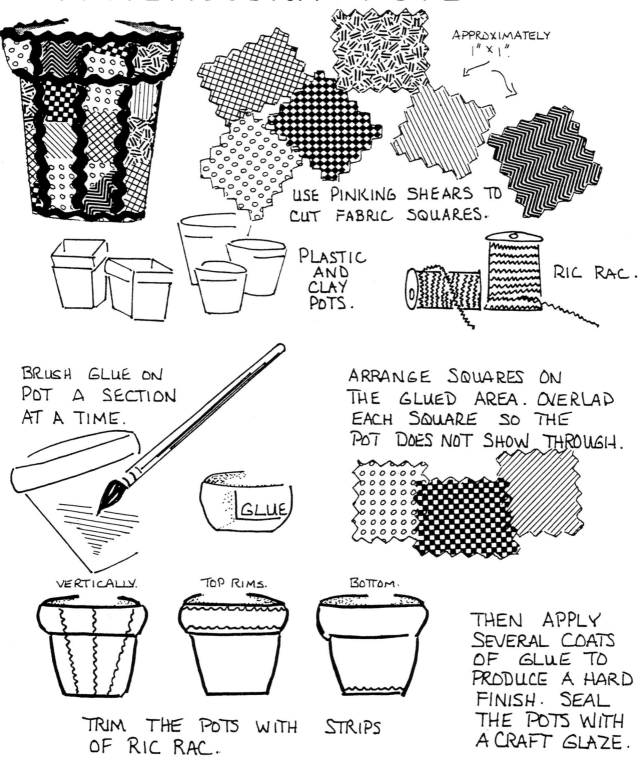

USE PINKING SHEARS TO CUT FABRIC SQUARES.

APPROXIMATELY 1" X 1".

PLASTIC AND CLAY POTS.

RIC RAC.

BRUSH GLUE ON POT A SECTION AT A TIME.

GLUE

ARRANGE SQUARES ON THE GLUED AREA. OVERLAP EACH SQUARE SO THE POT DOES NOT SHOW THROUGH.

VERTICALLY.

TOP RIMS.

BOTTOM.

TRIM THE POTS WITH OF RIC RAC.

STRIPS

THEN APPLY SEVERAL COATS OF GLUE TO PRODUCE A HARD FINISH. SEAL THE POTS WITH A CRAFT GLAZE.

WASTE BASKETS

Level of difficulty: *-*****

MATERIALS: Five-gallon ice cream cartons, fabric, craft glue, brushes, water, empty plastic containers, ric rac or other trim, pinking shears, plastic bags, varnish or craft glaze (optional).

APPLICATIONS: These waste baskets are an attractive addition to any room. Men seem to like this project because it is not dainty. Choose masculine prints.

PREPARATION BEFORE CRAFT SESSION: Using a pinking shears, cut strips of fabric 2 inches by 13 inches. Mix craft glue with water until it is the consistency of white glue.

CRAFT SESSION: Brush the glue on the empty container a section at a time. Arrange the strips of fabric attractively on the glue. You might like to place the strips diagonally across the container. Be certain to overlap each strip slightly so that the container will not show through the cloth. Then trim the basket with ric rac around the top and bottom edges. After the basket dries, apply several coats of the glue and water mixture over the entire container, letting it dry between each application. If you like, seal the basket with acrylic-based polyurethane. Do not use spray glazes, as the fumes are harmful.

WASTE BASKETS

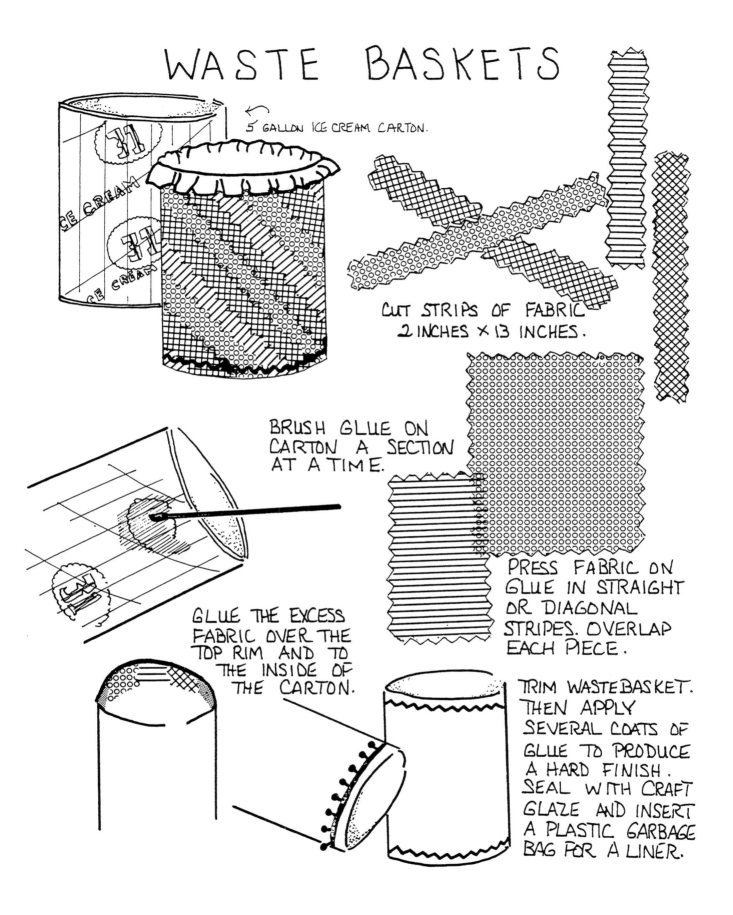

5 GALLON ICE CREAM CARTON.

CUT STRIPS OF FABRIC
2 INCHES × 13 INCHES.

BRUSH GLUE ON
CARTON A SECTION
AT A TIME.

PRESS FABRIC ON
GLUE IN STRAIGHT
OR DIAGONAL
STRIPES. OVERLAP
EACH PIECE.

GLUE THE EXCESS
FABRIC OVER THE
TOP RIM AND TO
THE INSIDE OF
THE CARTON.

TRIM WASTEBASKET.
THEN APPLY
SEVERAL COATS OF
GLUE TO PRODUCE
A HARD FINISH.
SEAL WITH CRAFT
GLAZE AND INSERT
A PLASTIC GARBAGE
BAG FOR A LINER.

CROSS STITCH

Level of difficulty: ***-*****

MATERIALS: Checked gingham, embroidery floss in a variety of colors, needles, scissors, thimble (optional), pencil, embroidery hoop or wooden frame, tacks, C-clamp.

APPLICATIONS: Many people look forward to senior years as a time to do creative stitchery. And then illness strikes and limits the use of an arm. The frame shown in the illustration can be anchored to a table top or wheelchair with a C-clamp so that a person with the use of only one arm can cross stitch. Use cross-stitch designs for aprons, towels, pillow cases, scarves, and pictures.

PREPARATION BEFORE CRAFT SESSION: Cut gingham into appropriate sizes for articles to be made. Finish the edges with a blanket stitch. Use large gingham print for those people who have difficulty seeing small squares. Using a pencil, prepare a design on the gingham. Then place the fabric in an embroidery hoop or secure it across a wooden frame with tacks. (Some people may prefer to create their own designs.)

CRAFT SESSION: Help each person choose an article to stitch and thread needles with appropriate colors. Then cross-stitch until the article is finished. Help knot and cut the thread. Perhaps the patient knows how to stitch initials on the completed article.

CROSS-STITCH

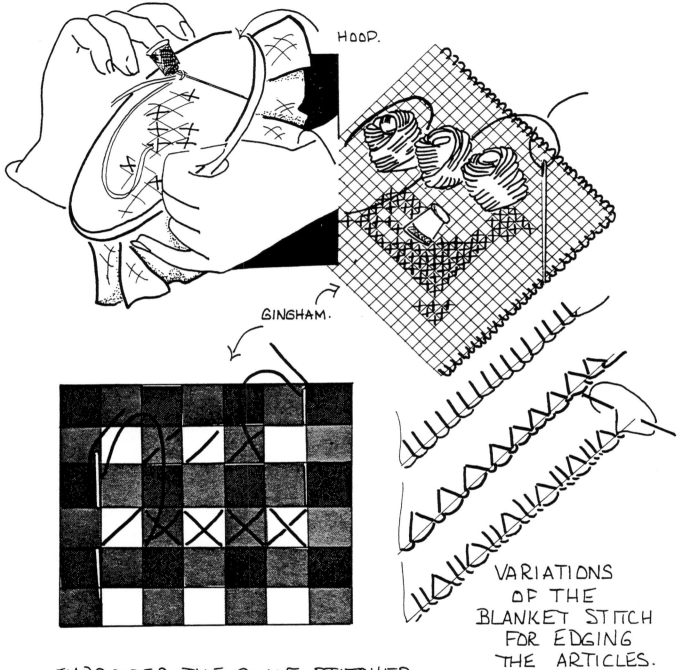

HOOP.

GINGHAM.

VARIATIONS
OF THE
BLANKET STITCH
FOR EDGING
THE ARTICLES.

EMBROIDER THE SLANT STITCHES
OF ONE ROW IN ONE DIRECTION.
THESE ARE CROSSED BY A SECOND
ROW OF STITCHES IN THE OPPOSITE.

CROSS-STITCH FRAME

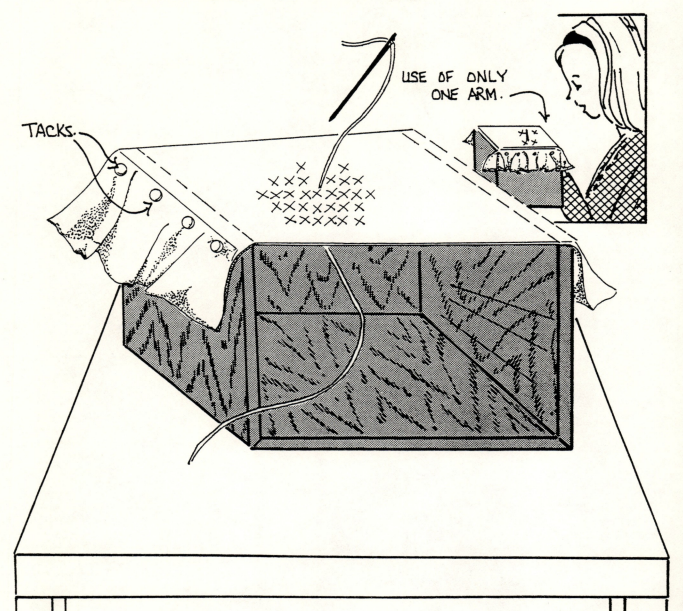

TACKS.

USE OF ONLY ONE ARM.

SEWING FRAME IS 4-SIDED WOODEN BOX. THE TOP AND FRONT ARE OPEN. SECURE CLOTH ACROSS TOP OPENING TIGHTLY WITH TACKS.

CROSS-STITCH PATTERN

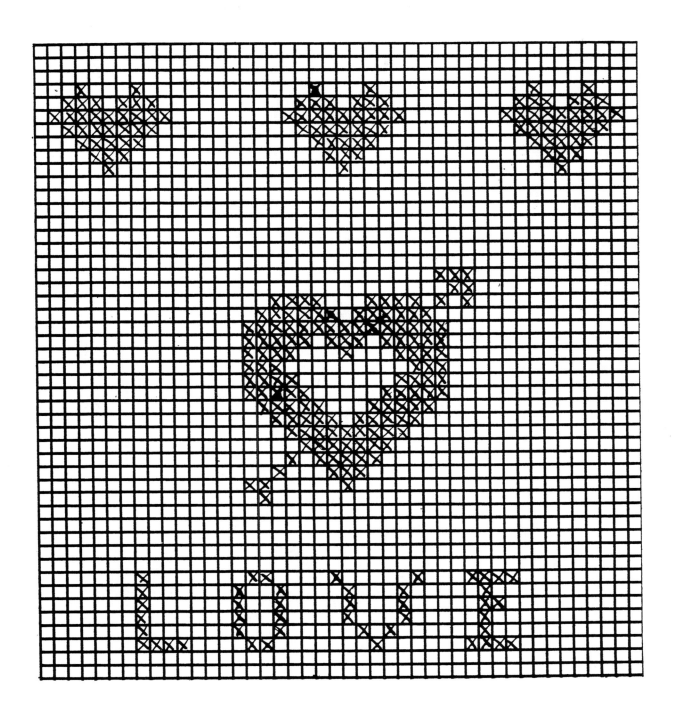

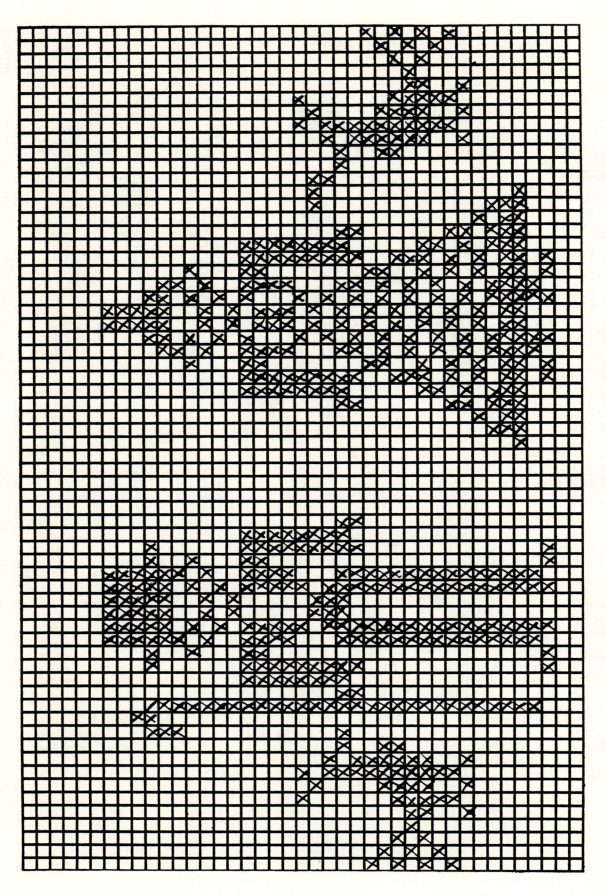

CROSS - STITCH PATTERN

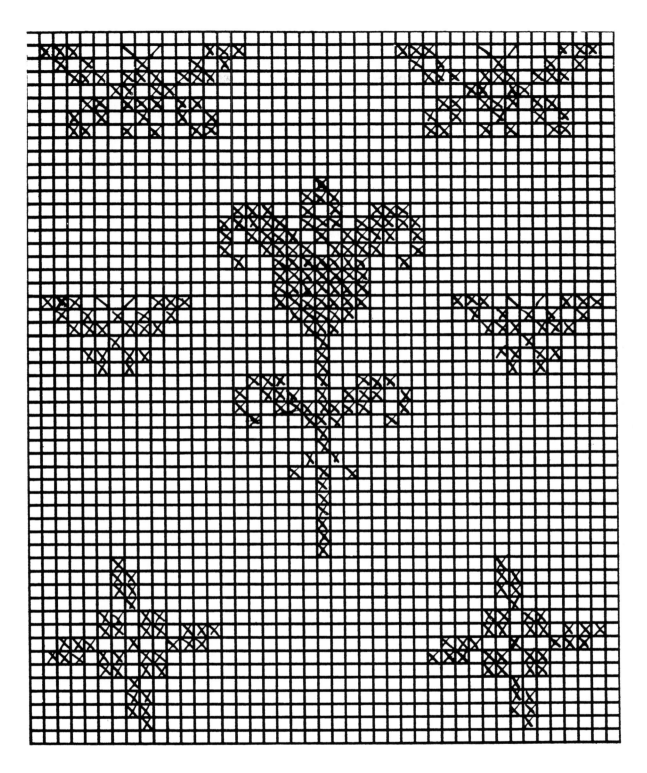

CROSS-STITCH PATTERN

Chapter Six

CRAFT PROJECTS FOR USE BY OTHER PATIENTS

MURALS

Level of difficulty: *-***

MATERIALS: Butcher paper, tempera paint, brushes, sponges, paper towels, water containers, markers, pastels, crayons, double-faced mounting tape, scissors, ruler, yardstick, glue stick, and dropcloths.

APPLICATIONS: Wall murals are nice to brighten hallways, common areas, and even individual patient rooms. They can be used as backdrops for plays, puppet shows, musical programs, and to announce special activities. They are also great party and holiday decorations.

PREPARATION BEFORE CRAFT SESSION: Measure and cut a length or two of butcher paper (depending on the desired height). If you choose to paint the mural on the wall, be certain to mount it low enough to accommodate wheelchairs. We recommend table-top production for more severely disabled patients. To keep the paper steady, you may secure it to the table top with glue stick. Select a theme and appropriate materials. You may want to predraw some areas of the mural design. Other projects in this book provide patterns and ideas.

CRAFT SESSION: Color the mural with paints, crayons, pastels, etc. Have participants sign the mural. Mount it after it has dried thoroughly.

MURALS

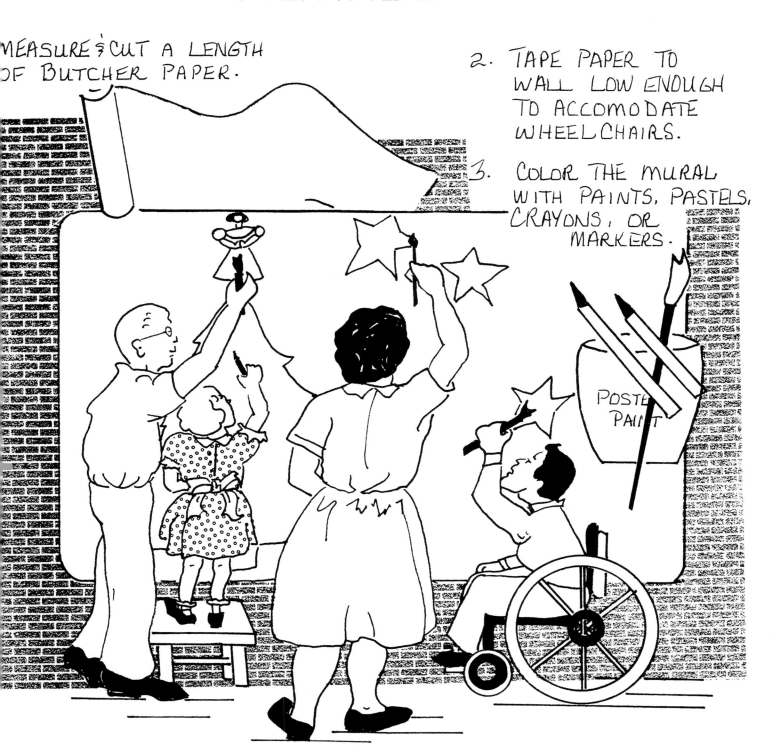

1. MEASURE & CUT A LENGTH OF BUTCHER PAPER.

2. TAPE PAPER TO WALL LOW ENOUGH TO ACCOMODATE WHEELCHAIRS.

3. COLOR THE MURAL WITH PAINTS, PASTELS, CRAYONS, OR MARKERS.

POSTER PAINT

4. MOUNT THE MURAL TO BRIGHTEN HALLWAYS, SHARE WITH PATIENTS, OR FOR PROGRAM PROPS.

MUSIC DAY

Level of difficulty: *-*****

MATERIALS: Tape player and pre-recorded music or an accompanist, hand made rhythm instruments, amplification system, overhead projector, sing-along sheets, and decorations.

APPLICATIONS: Music Days are almost always popular activities in any setting. The participants as well as the staff and other patients will enjoy the program. The patients may want to hold a "staff appreciation day." While some of the patients will not want to perform, their hand·made instruments and decorations will allow them to participate.

PREPARATION BEFORE CRAFT SESSION: Determine a theme such as "Western Day," "Golden Oldies," holiday themes, etc. Prepare decorations, invitations, decorated song sheets, and musical instruments, using other projects from this book. For example, we used "Wooden Horse" for Western Day. We also clipped the sing-along sheets in the horses' mouths and tied bright bandannas around the participants' necks.

CRAFT SESSION: Follow your program plan. You may want to have the staff nutritionist help you complete your theme with special refreshments. Patients often like to save decorations and instruments as souvenirs.

MUSIC DAY

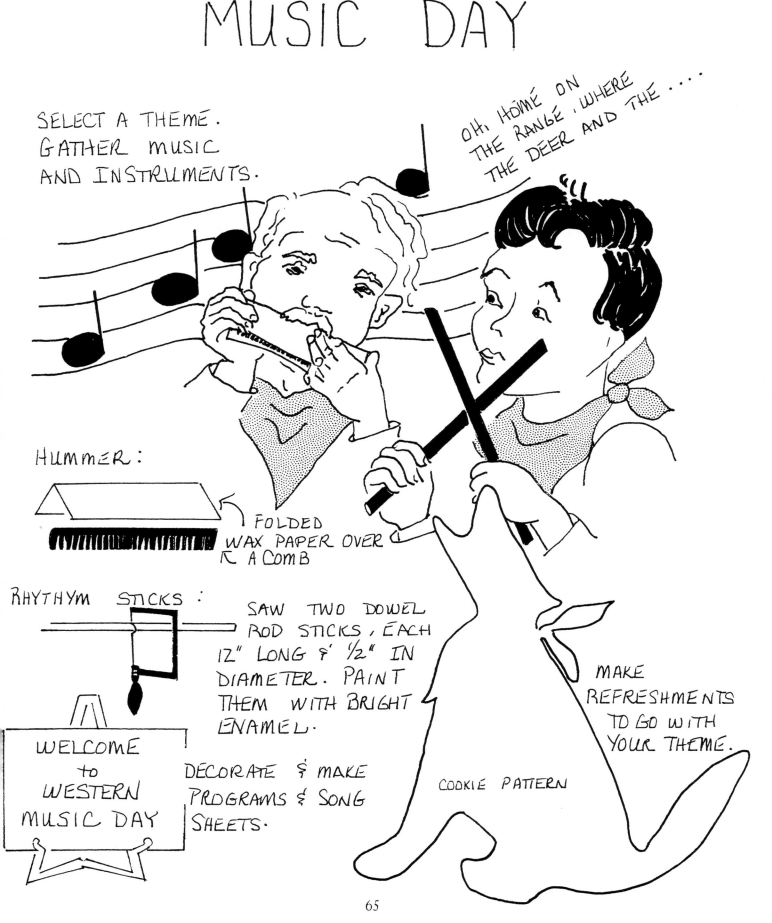

SELECT A THEME. GATHER MUSIC AND INSTRUMENTS.

OH, HOME ON THE RANGE, WHERE THE DEER AND THE . . . .

Hummer:

FOLDED WAX PAPER OVER A COMB

RHYTHYM STICKS:

SAW TWO DOWEL ROD STICKS, EACH 12" LONG & 1/2" IN DIAMETER. PAINT THEM WITH BRIGHT ENAMEL.

WELCOME to WESTERN MUSIC DAY

DECORATE & MAKE PROGRAMS & SONG SHEETS.

COOKIE PATTERN

MAKE REFRESHMENTS TO GO WITH YOUR THEME.

DECORATED WALKING STICKS

Level of difficulty: ***-*****

MATERIALS: Smooth branches or limbs about 4 feet in length, acrylic paints, brushes, newspaper or white adhesive tape, felt marking pens in a variety of colors.

APPLICATIONS: Many people enjoy using a walking stick when strolling through the garden, around corridors, or on field trips to shopping centers or special events.

PREPARATION BEFORE CRAFT SESSION: Prepare some branches for those who find paints too messy. To do this, wrap adhesive tape around sections of the branches. You will be able to see the colors of the pens on these white areas. Some may prefer to glue fabric strips on the branches rather than tape.

CRAFT SESSION: Place the branches over newspaper and make designs with paints. Try using a knot as a nose of a face. Use felt marking pens to color the adhesive tape, if you do not like to work with paint.

DECORATED WALKING STICKS

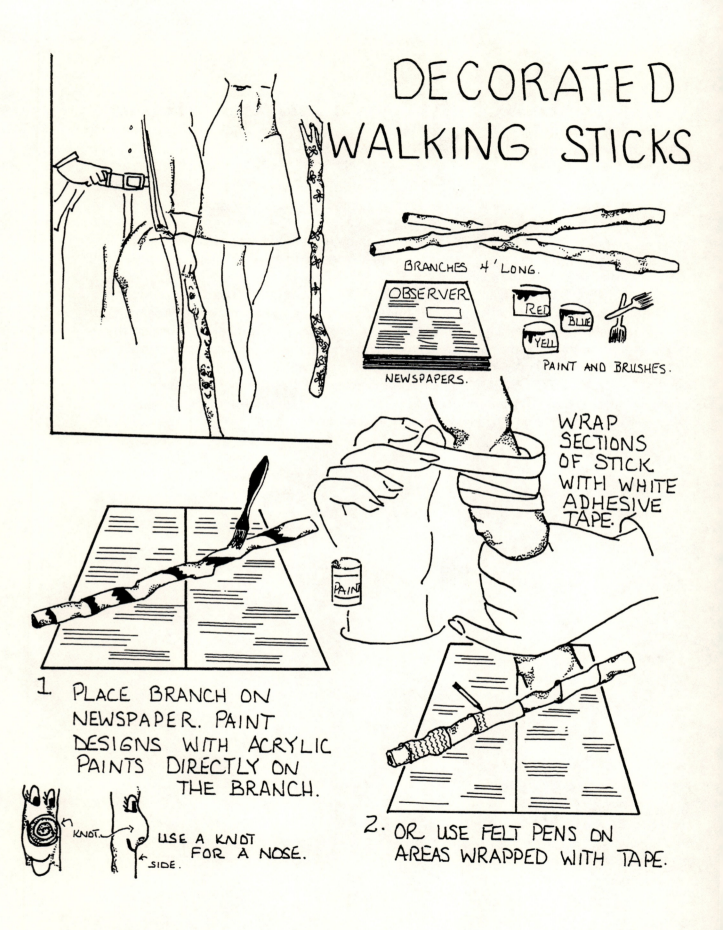

BRANCHES 4' LONG.

OBSERVER

NEWSPAPERS.

RED
BLUE
YELL

PAINT AND BRUSHES.

PAINT

WRAP SECTIONS OF STICK WITH WHITE ADHESIVE TAPE.

1. PLACE BRANCH ON NEWSPAPER. PAINT DESIGNS WITH ACRYLIC PAINTS DIRECTLY ON THE BRANCH.

KNOT.

USE A KNOT FOR A NOSE.

SIDE.

2. OR USE FELT PENS ON AREAS WRAPPED WITH TAPE.

IDEAS FOR DECORATED WALKING STICK

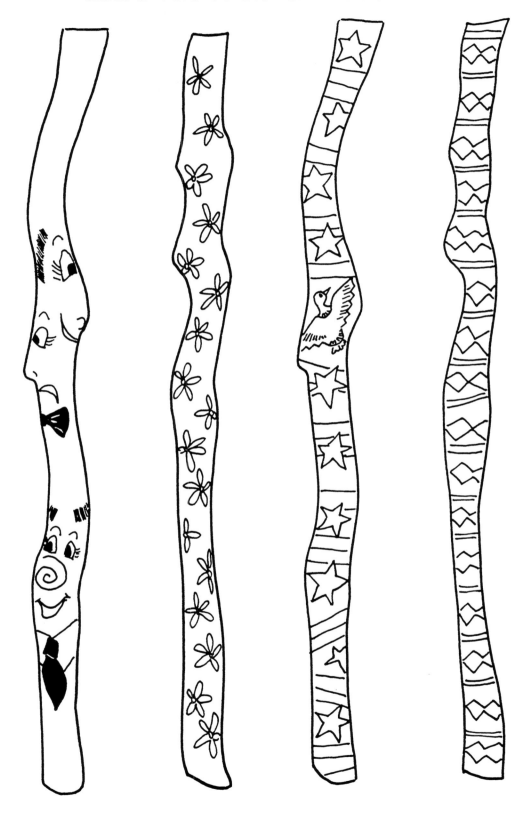

PILLOWS

Level of difficulty: *-*****

MATERIALS: Fabric scraps, scissors, needle, thread, stuffing, several large sheets of paper, pencil, iron, ironing board, pins.

APPLICATIONS: Throw pillows are good for back support in wheelchairs or neck support in beds. Try making thin pillows for cushions to sit upon. It is nice to have those who can sew well make the pillow covers and let senile or blind patients then stuff the pillows. Choose fabrics you think friends would enjoy.

PREPARATION BEFORE CRAFT SESSION: Make paper patterns for the pillows. You can make rectangles, squares, circles, or animal shapes. Pin the pattern to the fabric, and cut out two pieces of cloth the same shape and size. Press the fabric pieces with a warm iron. Be sure to keep the cord and iron away from patients.

CRAFT SESSION: Place the front of the pillow, design face up, on a table and lay the pillow back on top, making certain that all the sides and corners match as exactly as possible. Be sure that the wrong side of each piece of fabric is on the outside, as you will be turning the pillow inside out. Pin the two pieces of cloth securely together. Using a needle and thread, stitch around the pillow about $5/8$ inch from the edge, leaving a 6-inch opening for the stuffing. Clip any corners close to the stitching as shown in the illustration. Remove the pins. Then turn the pillow inside out. Poke the corners out until the shape is accurate again. Stuff the pillow, being sure to push the stuffing (polyester, cotton, old nylons, or fabric bits) into the corners. Fill the pillow as full as you like; then pin the opening closed and sew it by hand. Shake the pillow to distribute the stuffing evenly.

PILLOWS

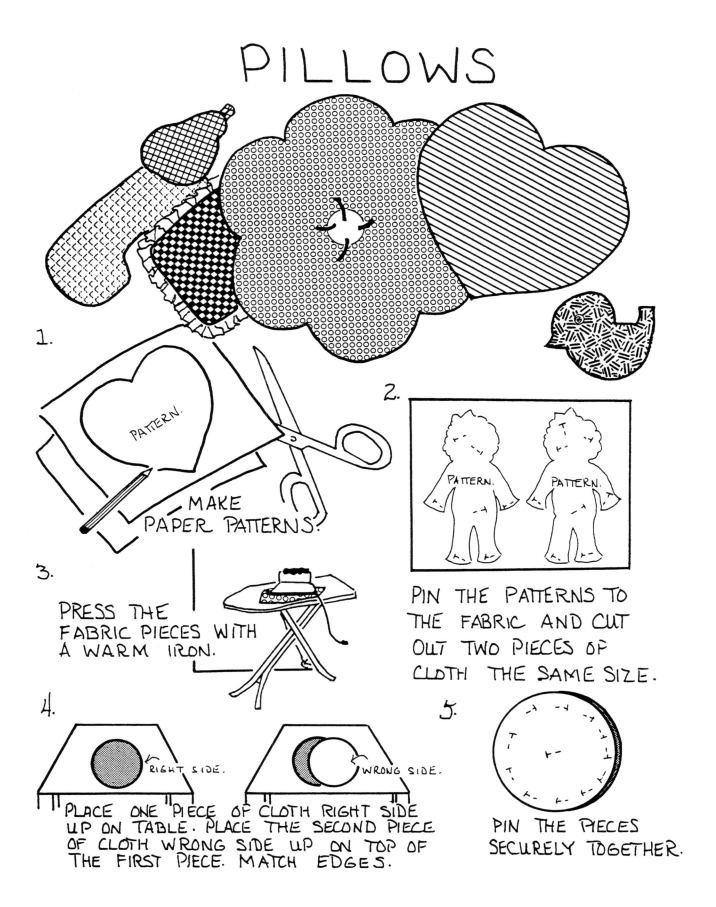

1. MAKE PAPER PATTERNS.

2. PIN THE PATTERNS TO THE FABRIC AND CUT OUT TWO PIECES OF CLOTH THE SAME SIZE.

3. PRESS THE FABRIC PIECES WITH A WARM IRON.

4. RIGHT SIDE. WRONG SIDE. PLACE ONE PIECE OF CLOTH RIGHT SIDE UP ON TABLE. PLACE THE SECOND PIECE OF CLOTH WRONG SIDE UP ON TOP OF THE FIRST PIECE. MATCH EDGES.

5. PIN THE PIECES SECURELY TOGETHER.

PILLOWS

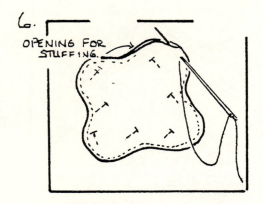

OPENING FOR STUFFING.

STITCH AROUND THE PILLOW ABOUT 5/8 INCH FROM THE EDGE, LEAVING A 6 INCH OPENING.

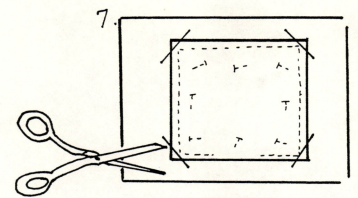

CLIP CORNERS CLOSE TO THE STITCHING. REMOVE THE PINS.

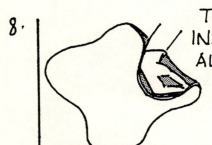

TURN THE PILLOW INSIDE OUT. POKE ALL THE CORNERS TO SHAPE THE PILLOW.

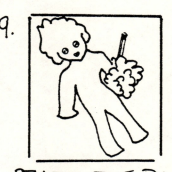

STUFF THE PILLOW. BE SURE TO GET INTO ALL THE CORNERS.

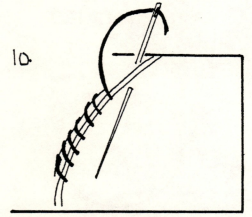

PIN THE OPENING AND SEW IT CLOSED.

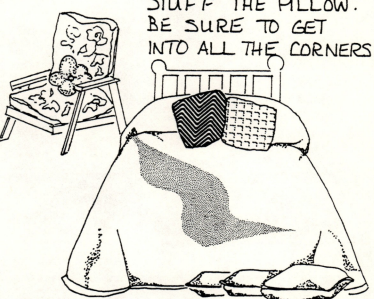

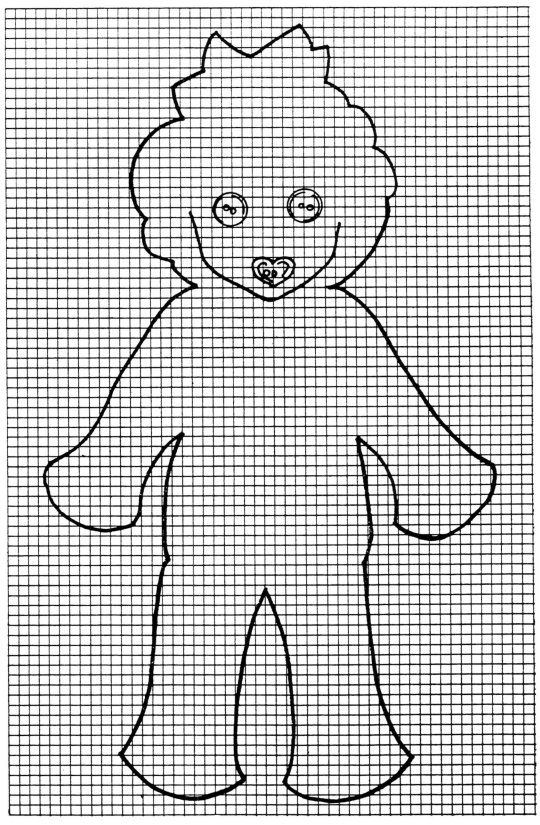

ENLARGE THIS PILLOW PATTERN.

HANGING BASKET

Level of difficulty: ****_*****

MATERIALS: Raffia or twine, buttons or beads, metal rings, scissors, cup hook or bracket.

APPLICATIONS: This hanging basket is like a large net and will hold different shapes and sizes of containers for plants and flowers. A basket makes an especially nice gift for a friend who does not have enough table space to display his plants.

PREPARATION BEFORE CRAFT SESSION: Cut raffia or twine into 48-inch lengths. Fasten eight or twelve lengths of raffia to a metal or bone ring as shown in the illustration.

CRAFT SESSION: Start weaving at the bottom of the basket. To do this, take one end of the raffia loop and one end of the loop next to it. String these through a button or bead until they are about 2 inches from the ring. String the next row of buttons with the opposite raffia lengths 3 inches from the first row of buttons. Repeat another row 3 inches farther on the raffia; and, if you wish the basket still larger, add another row. Tie all the ends to hold them together at the top. Hook this hanger over a cup hook or bracket.

HANGING BASKET

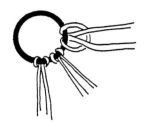

FASTEN 8 OR 12 LENGTHS OF RAFFIA TO A METAL RING. RAFFIA FOLDED SHOULD BE 24".

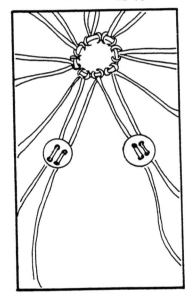

TAKE ONE END OF ONE RAFFIA LOOP AND ONE END OF THE LOOP NEXT TO IT. STRING THESE THROUGH A BUTTON 2" FROM THE RING. CONTINUE AROUND THE RING.

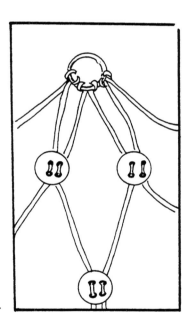

THEN STRING THE NEXT ROW OF BUTTONS WITH THE OPPOSITE RAFFIA LENGTHS 3" FROM THE FIRST ROW OF BUTTONS.

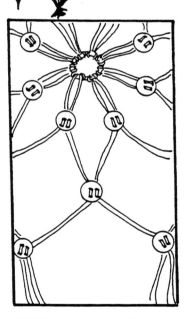

REPEAT ANOTHER ROW 3" FARTHER ON THE RAFFIA.

WIND CHIMES

Level of difficulty: ***-*****

MATERIALS: Round-headed clothespins, plastic lids, ribbon colored string, scissors, nail, cup hook.

APPLICATIONS: Musical wind chimes which sing in the breeze are a welcome addition to any patio area. Try hanging the chimes over an open window. Bed ridden patients like to watch the movement and hear the music of the wind chimes.

PREPARATION BEFORE CRAFT SESSION: Using a nail, punch ten pairs of holes in a plastic lid about 1 inch apart as shown in the illustration. Cut ten 15-inch pieces of string for each lid.

CRAFT SESSION: Push a piece of string up through one hole in the lid and down through the other. Make a knot in the end of the string too large to pull back through the hole. Pull the string tightly. Tie the other end of the string around the neck of a clothespin. Repeat this process until there are ten clothespins hanging about the same height from the lid. Then poke a hole in the center of the lid and tie a pretty ribbon through it for hanging the chimes from a cup hook.

WIND CHIMES

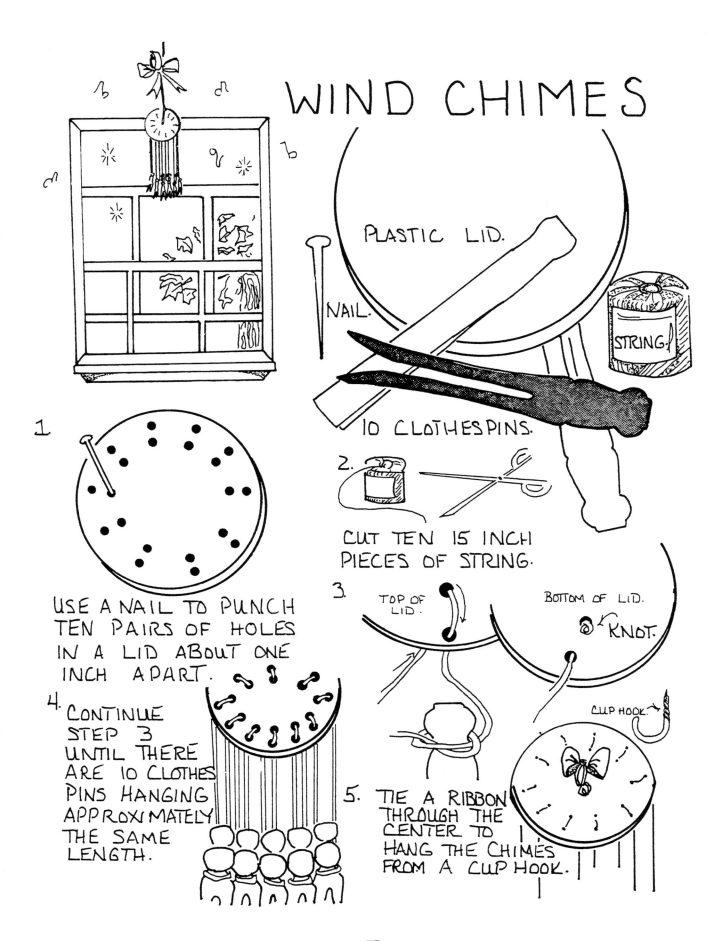

PLASTIC LID.

NAIL.

STRING!

10 CLOTHESPINS.

2. CUT TEN 15 INCH PIECES OF STRING.

1. USE A NAIL TO PUNCH TEN PAIRS OF HOLES IN A LID ABOUT ONE INCH APART.

3. TOP OF LID. BOTTOM OF LID. KNOT.

CUP HOOK.

4. CONTINUE STEP 3 UNTIL THERE ARE 10 CLOTHES PINS HANGING APPROXIMATELY THE SAME LENGTH.

5. TIE A RIBBON THROUGH THE CENTER TO HANG THE CHIMES FROM A CUP HOOK.

PAPER FLOWERS

Level of difficulty: *

MATERIALS: Colored tissue paper, scissors, floral wire cut in 16-inch lengths.

APPLICATIONS: These festive flowers brighten any room when put in a vase or taped to the wall. It is nice to give the flowers to nonambulatory friends on their birthdays or as get well wishes. The flowers may also be used for stage decorations for music programs or special presentations.

PREPARATION BEFORE CRAFT SESSION: Cut the pieces of tissue in half to make pieces approximately 15 inches by 20 inches. They do not have to be exact. Then stack two or three pieces of tissue in the same or varied colors and fold to make a paper fan. Tie each fan in the center with a piece of floral wire. Make dozens.

CRAFT SESSION: Separate the layers of tissue paper on both sides of the wire. The ruffled paper will now look like frilly flower petals.

PAPER FLOWERS

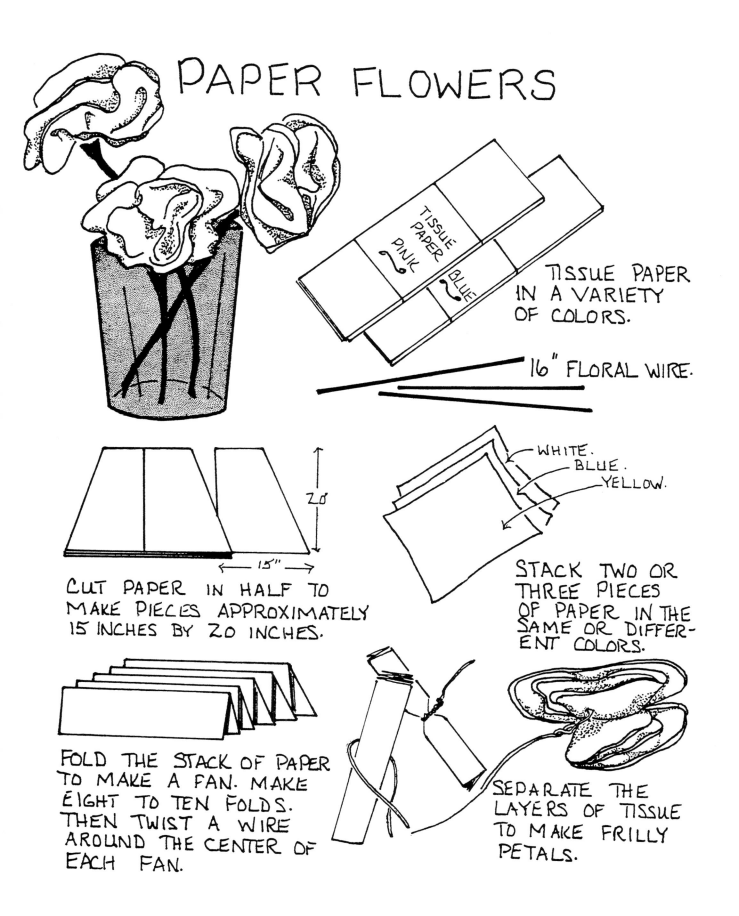

TISSUE PAPER
PINK
BLUE

TISSUE PAPER
IN A VARIETY
OF COLORS.

16" FLORAL WIRE.

20

15"

CUT PAPER IN HALF TO
MAKE PIECES APPROXIMATELY
15 INCHES BY 20 INCHES.

WHITE.
BLUE.
YELLOW.

STACK TWO OR
THREE PIECES
OF PAPER IN THE
SAME OR DIFFER-
ENT COLORS.

FOLD THE STACK OF PAPER
TO MAKE A FAN. MAKE
EIGHT TO TEN FOLDS.
THEN TWIST A WIRE
AROUND THE CENTER OF
EACH FAN.

SEPARATE THE
LAYERS OF TISSUE
TO MAKE FRILLY
PETALS.

79

MOBILES

Level of difficulty: **-*****

MATERIALS: White drawing paper, black felt marking pen, wax paper, colored tissue paper, nylon thread, iron, 12-inch stick or dowel or wire from a coat hanger, glue stick, scissors, needle, thumbtacks.

APPLICATIONS: Mobiles have attracted the eyes of children and adults for centuries. These colorful butterflies shimmer with changing patterns when hung from a ceiling. Share the mobiles with nonambulatory patients.

PREPARATION BEFORE CRAFT SESSION: Using a black pen, trace five butterfly patterns on each piece of white drawing paper. Leave about 2 inches between each butterfly. Use glue stick to secure the papers to the table in front of each person. Then use the glue stick again to cover each piece of drawing paper with a piece of wax paper.

CRAFT SESSION: Arrange scraps of colored tissue paper on the wax paper to look like butterflies. The patterns on the drawing paper will help, but remember that the butterflies do not have to be perfect. Carefully place the other piece of wax paper over the tissue paper scraps. Press with a warm iron. Be sure no patients are near the warm iron or its cord.

This process will seal the designs between the wax papers. Cut out the butterflies leaving 1/4 inch border of wax paper around each one. Using nylon thread and a needle to puncture the wax paper, tie five butterflies to each stick or wire. Tie one or two pieces of thread to the stick to hang the completed mobile from the ceiling with thumbtacks. If cost is not a consideration, substitute laminating acetate or clear contact paper for the wax paper.

MOBILES

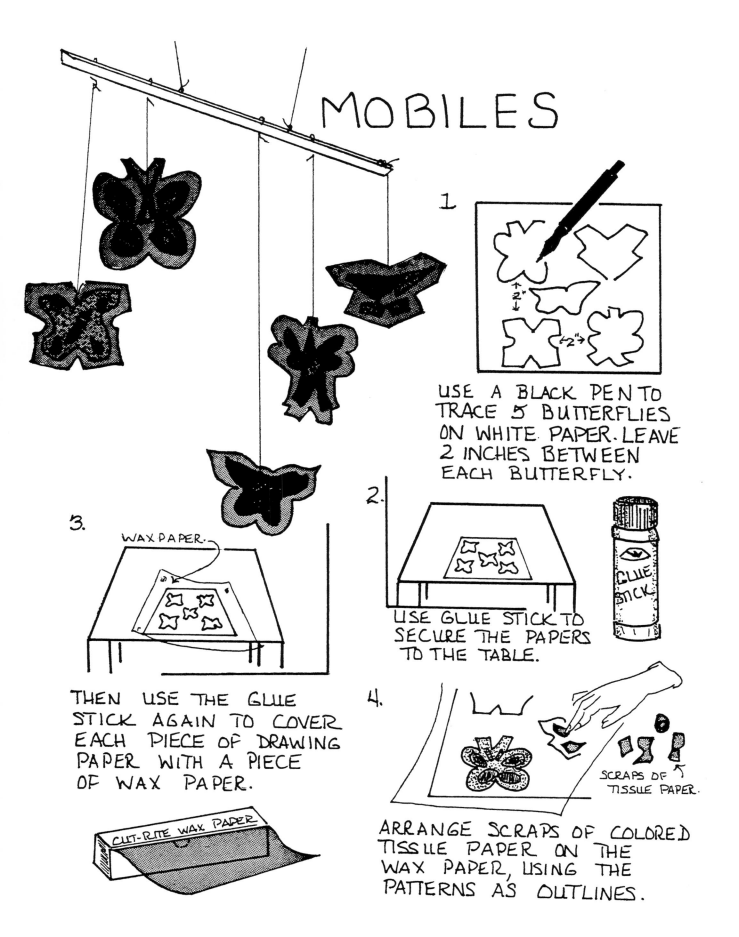

1

USE A BLACK PEN TO
TRACE 5 BUTTERFLIES
ON WHITE PAPER. LEAVE
2 INCHES BETWEEN
EACH BUTTERFLY.

2.

USE GLUE STICK TO
SECURE THE PAPERS
TO THE TABLE.

GLUE
STICK

3.

WAX PAPER.

THEN USE THE GLUE
STICK AGAIN TO COVER
EACH PIECE OF DRAWING
PAPER WITH A PIECE
OF WAX PAPER.

CUT-RITE WAX PAPER

4.

SCRAPS OF
TISSUE PAPER.

ARRANGE SCRAPS OF COLORED
TISSUE PAPER ON THE
WAX PAPER, USING THE
PATTERNS AS OUTLINES.

MOBILES

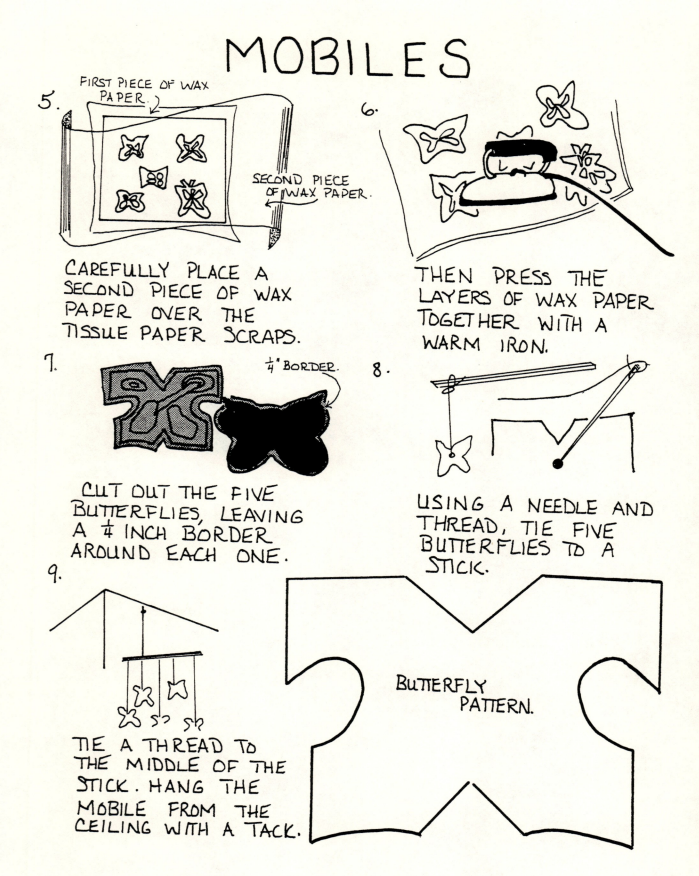

5. FIRST PIECE OF WAX PAPER.

SECOND PIECE OF WAX PAPER.

CAREFULLY PLACE A SECOND PIECE OF WAX PAPER OVER THE TISSUE PAPER SCRAPS.

6. THEN PRESS THE LAYERS OF WAX PAPER TOGETHER WITH A WARM IRON.

7. ¼" BORDER.

CUT OUT THE FIVE BUTTERFLIES, LEAVING A ¼ INCH BORDER AROUND EACH ONE.

8. USING A NEEDLE AND THREAD, TIE FIVE BUTTERFLIES TO A STICK.

9. TIE A THREAD TO THE MIDDLE OF THE STICK. HANG THE MOBILE FROM THE CEILING WITH A TACK.

BUTTERFLY PATTERN.

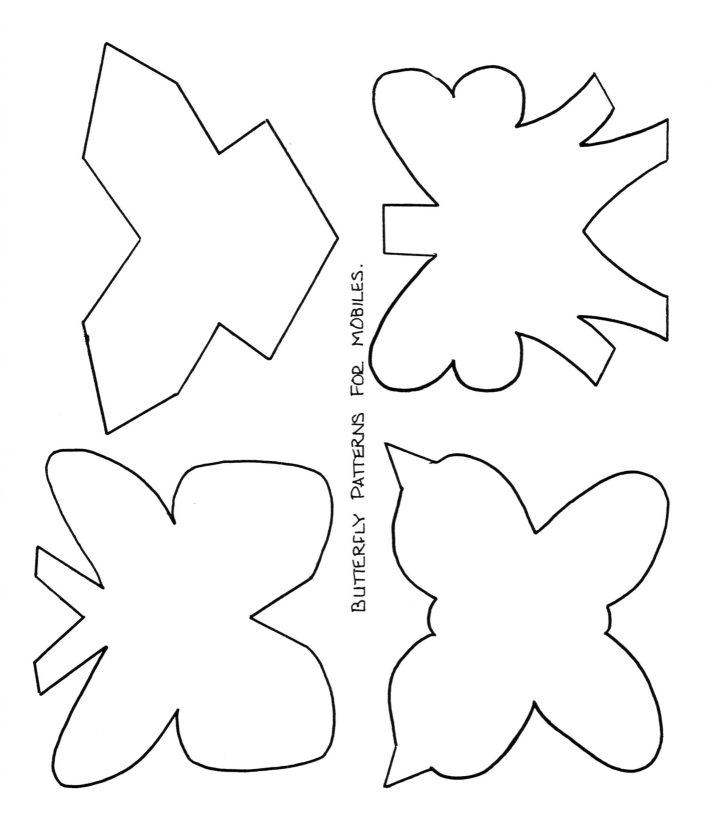

BUTTERFLY PATTERNS FOR MOBILES.

SPRING PLANT-IN

Level of difficulty: **-*****

MATERIALS: Plastic or clay flower pots, contact paper, scissors, newspaper, water, potting soil, seeds.

APPLICATIONS: In the springtime, thoughts turn to nature. Let each person who is able, plant and decorate a flower pot. Then put all the pots together along the walkways of your building or in a central patio. Let ambulatory patients be in charge of watering the pots. Everyone can enjoy the blossoms. Nurseries will be happy to donate old pots, or use gallon size plastic food containers with holes punched in the bottoms for drainage.

PREPARATION BEFORE CRAFT SESSION: None.

CRAFT SESSION: Cut flowers out of contact paper. Peel off the backing, and stick the contact paper flowers on the pots for decoration. Spread newspapers to catch dirt. Fill the pots with soil. Plant the seeds and water them. Place the pots outside in an easy-to-see location.

SPRING PLANT-IN

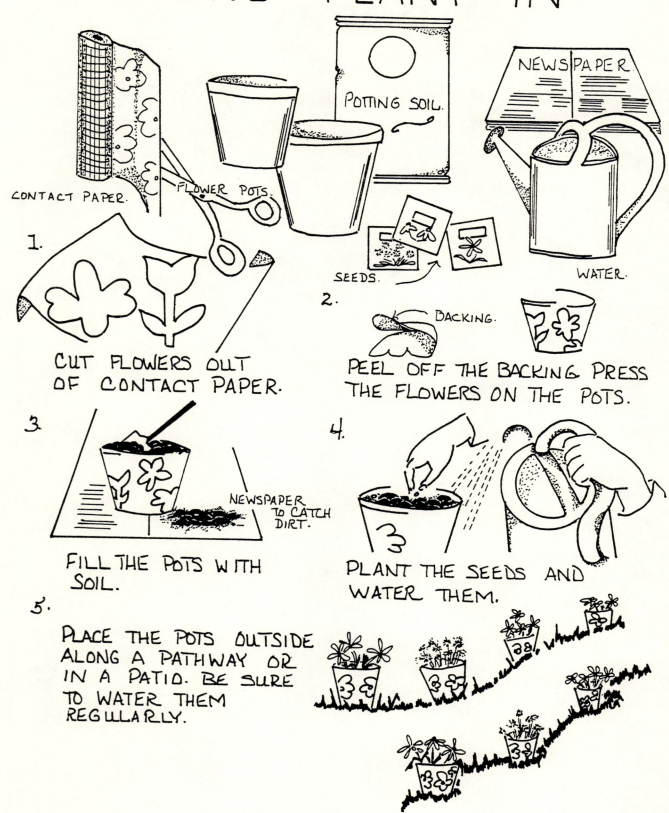

CONTACT PAPER.

FLOWER POTS

POTTING SOIL.

NEWSPAPER

SEEDS.

WATER.

1. CUT FLOWERS OUT OF CONTACT PAPER.

2. BACKING.
PEEL OFF THE BACKING PRESS THE FLOWERS ON THE POTS.

3. NEWSPAPER TO CATCH DIRT.
FILL THE POTS WITH SOIL.

4. PLANT THE SEEDS AND WATER THEM.

5. PLACE THE POTS OUTSIDE ALONG A PATHWAY OR IN A PATIO. BE SURE TO WATER THEM REGULARLY.

PATTERNS FOR FLOWER CUT-OUTS

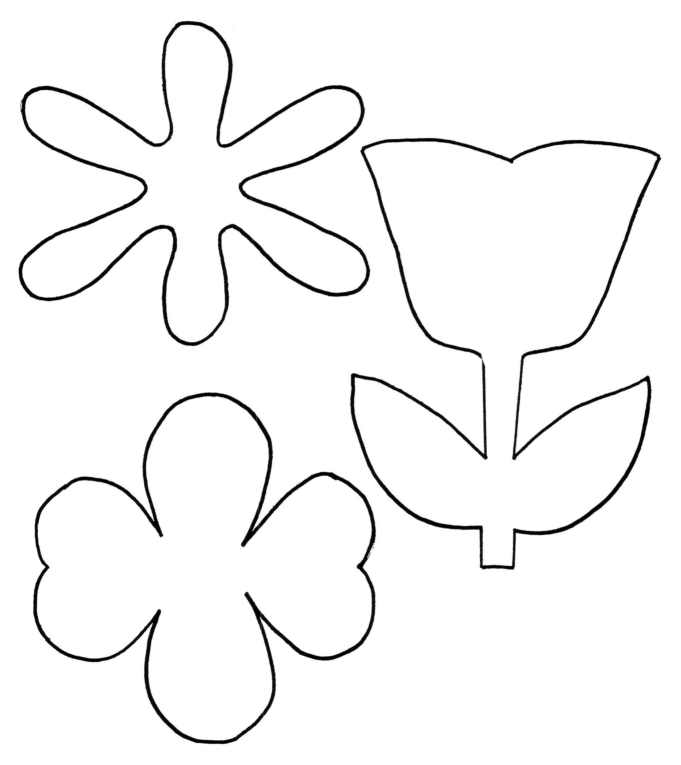

GREETING CARD HOLDERS

Level of difficulty: ❋❋

MATERIALS: 46-ounce juice cans, yarn, scissors.

APPLICATIONS: The card holder is nice to hold get-well cards on a dresser or night stand. Use red and green yarn for Christmas or pink and blue yarn for a baby shower gift.

PREPARATION BEFORE CRAFT SESSION: Wash cans and cut out both ends of each can. Loop the yarn through the can and tie a knot to secure the yarn.

CRAFT SESSION: Have each person wind the yarn through the can over and over again until the entire can is covered with yarn. It is best to pull the yarn as tight as possible. When the can is covered with yarn, help each person cut and knot the yarn on the inside of the can. The holder is now ready to have cards inserted.

GREETING CARD HOLDERS

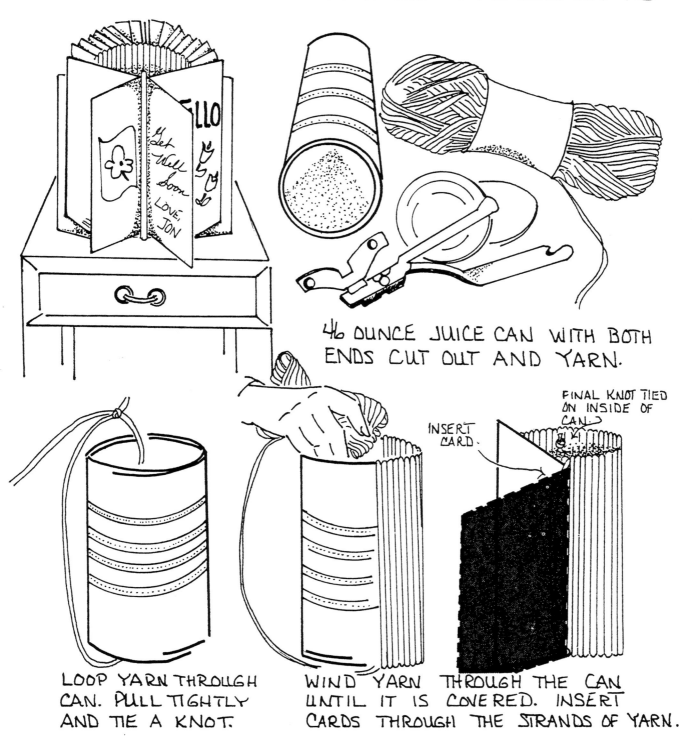

46 OUNCE JUICE CAN WITH BOTH ENDS CUT OUT AND YARN.

INSERT CARD.

FINAL KNOT TIED ON INSIDE OF CAN.

LOOP YARN THROUGH CAN. PULL TIGHTLY AND TIE A KNOT.

WIND YARN THROUGH THE CAN UNTIL IT IS COVERED. INSERT CARDS THROUGH THE STRANDS OF YARN.

BEDSIDE RACKS

Level of difficulty: *

MATERIALS: 46 ounce juice cans, fabric, pinking shears, glue, ribbon.

APPLICATIONS: The bedside rack is nice to hold magazines or tissues. Tie the racks with the ribbon to headboards or the inside of bed rails for patients who cannot reach their night stands.

PREPARATION BEFORE CRAFT SESSION: Wash cans and cut out both ends of each can. Cut ribbon into 36-inch lengths. Cut fabric with pinking shears into pieces 7¼ inches by 13½ inches.

CRAFT SESSION: Glue the fabric to the can. Loop the ribbon through the can and tie a bow.

BEDSIDE RACKS

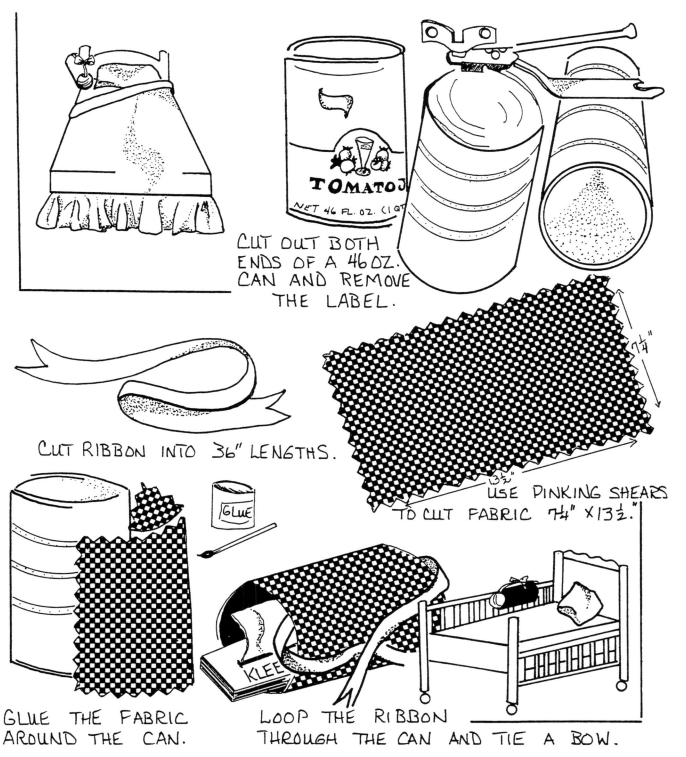

CUT OUT BOTH ENDS OF A 46 OZ. CAN AND REMOVE THE LABEL.

CUT RIBBON INTO 36" LENGTHS.

USE PINKING SHEARS TO CUT FABRIC 7¼" × 13½."

GLUE THE FABRIC AROUND THE CAN.

LOOP THE RIBBON THROUGH THE CAN AND TIE A BOW.

EASTER CENTERPIECES

Level of difficulty: *-***

MATERIALS: Yellow construction paper, scissors, glue, felt marking pens or crayons, paper plates, small candy eggs, cellophane grass, glue stick.

APPLICATIONS: These easy-to-make holiday centerpieces are nice to brighten a bleak room of a nonambulatory patient. Also, make many centerpieces and use them to decorate the dining-hall tables of your home or institution. Be careful that candy eggs are not in the reach of diabetics. You may prefer to substitute plastic eggs.

PREPARATION BEFORE CRAFT SESSION: Trace two patterns of each figure and cut them out of yellow construction paper. Note the illustration. Using glue stick, secure two patterns of each figure facing each other in front of each person. There will be a total of six cutouts for each centerpiece.

CRAFT SESSION: Color the cutouts with pens or crayons. Spread glue near the top on the back of each figure, and paste them together; the bottom part is not pasted, as it spreads apart. Fold the bases outward, each side in an opposite direction. Then spread glue on the bottom of the base of each figure, and paste the three figures on a paper plate. Arrange cellophane grass and eggs between and around the figures.

EASTER CENTERPIECES

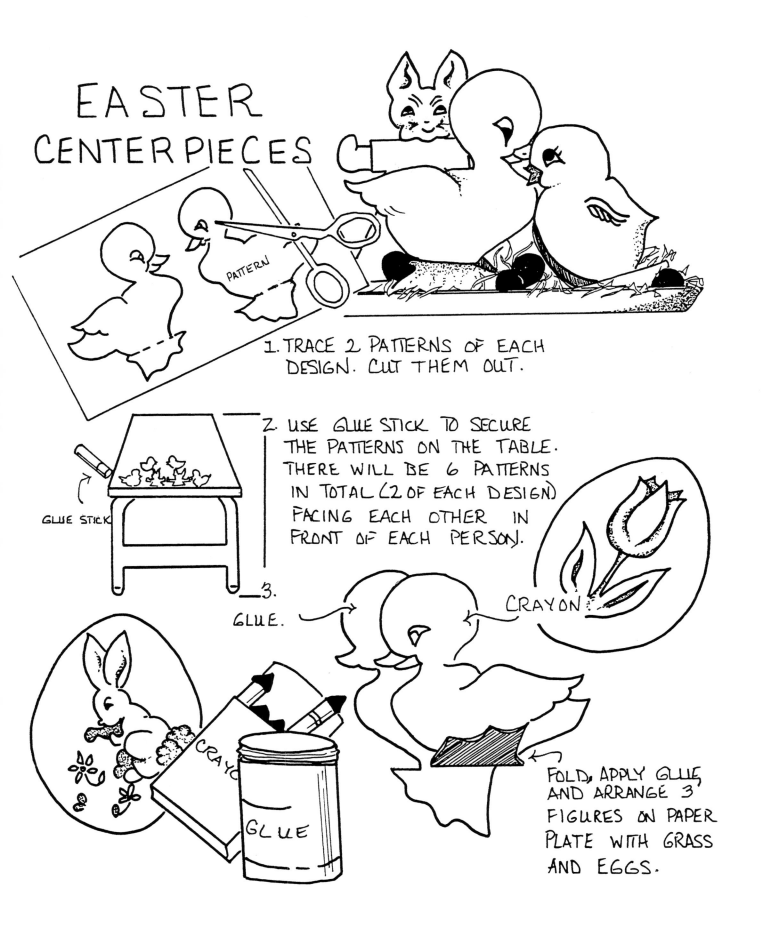

PATTERN

1. TRACE 2 PATTERNS OF EACH DESIGN. CUT THEM OUT.

GLUE STICK

2. USE GLUE STICK TO SECURE THE PATTERNS ON THE TABLE. THERE WILL BE 6 PATTERNS IN TOTAL (2 OF EACH DESIGN) FACING EACH OTHER IN FRONT OF EACH PERSON.

3. GLUE.

CRAYON

CRAYO

GLUE

FOLD, APPLY GLUE, AND ARRANGE 3 FIGURES ON PAPER PLATE WITH GRASS AND EGGS.

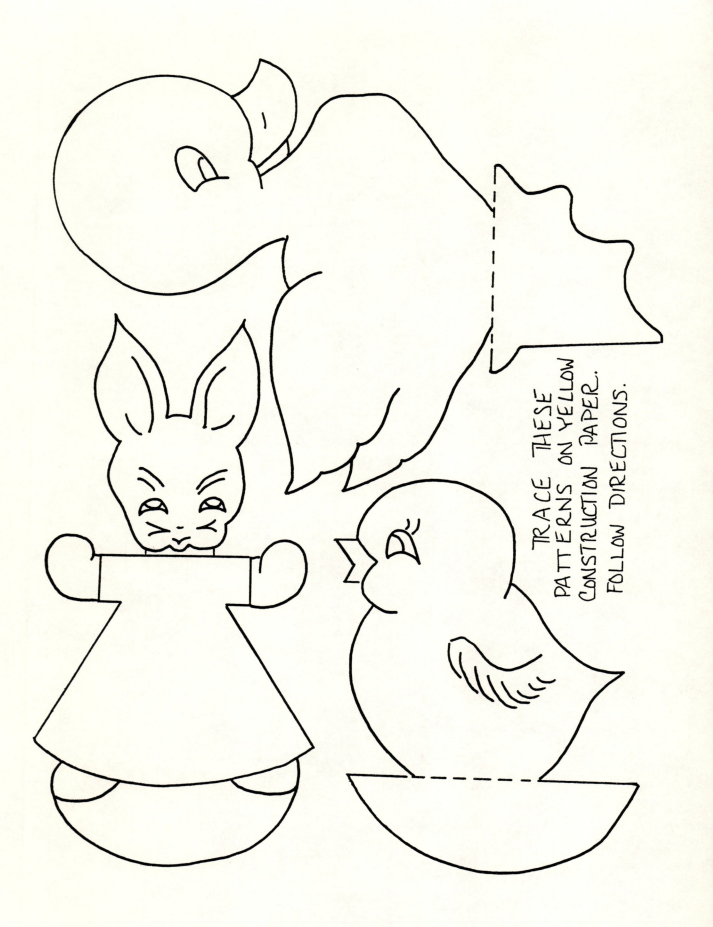

TRACE THESE PATTERNS ON YELLOW CONSTRUCTION PAPER. FOLLOW DIRECTIONS.

Chapter Seven

CRAFT PROJECTS TO GIVE TO FAMILY MEMBERS

PHOTO PUZZLES

Level of difficulty: **-*****

MATERIALS: A Polaroid® camera and film, copier, scissors, glue stick, graphite or carbon paper, construction paper or light weight poster board, puzzle pattern, masking tape, colored pencils, ball point pens, envelopes.

APPLICATIONS: These unique puzzles make happy gifts for family and friends.

PREPARATION BEFORE CRAFT SESSION: Take a photograph of each participant. You may want a seasonal theme such as a picture taken with Santa or the Easter Bunny. A local church or civic organization may have volunteer Bunnies, Santas, clowns, etc. Enlarge the photos to puzzle size. Draw a puzzle pattern to fit the puzzle size, and cut the construction paper and graphite or carbon paper to the same size. Be sure to use fewer pieces within your pattern to decrease the level of difficulty for the more disabled participants. You can incorporate seasonal shapes within your pattern; for example, hearts, ornaments and fall leaves. You will need one pattern for each participant.

CRAFT SESSION: Color the images with colored pencils if using black and white copies. Coat the back of the image with glue. Be certain to coat the entire surface, and then secure it to the construction paper. Assist the participants in assembling the photo, carbon paper, and pattern. The photo should be on the table, face-up; the carbon should be face-down on the photo; the pattern should be placed on top, face-up. Tape the top and bottom edges of your stack to the table surface for stabilization. Have the participants firmly trace the pattern with a ball point pen. Remove the pattern and carbon paper. Cut out the puzzle pieces. Package it in a pretty envelope. (See potato print cards for an envelope pattern.)

PHOTO PUZZLES

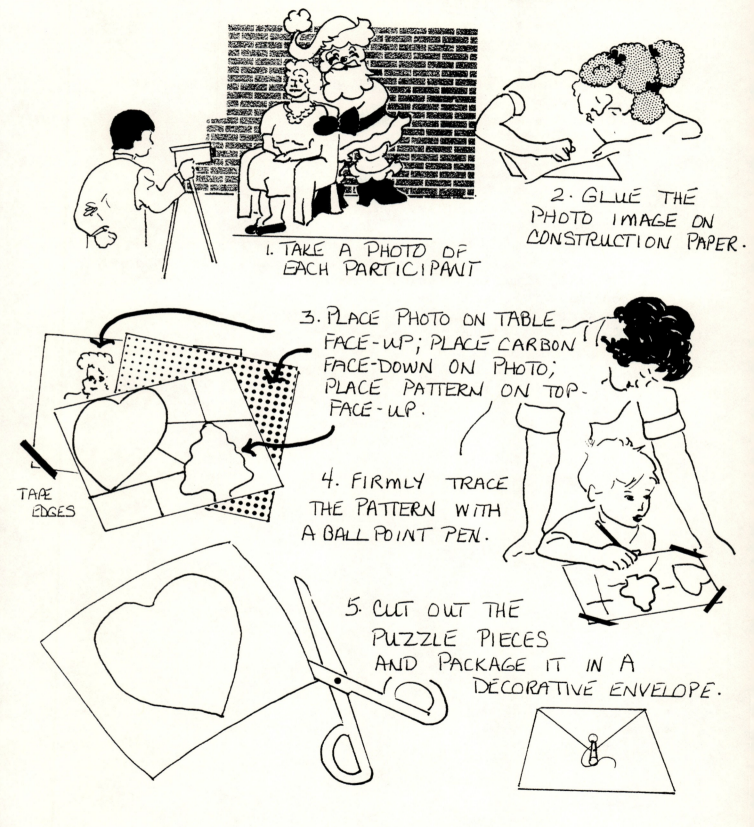

1. TAKE A PHOTO OF EACH PARTICIPANT

2. GLUE THE PHOTO IMAGE ON CONSTRUCTION PAPER.

3. PLACE PHOTO ON TABLE FACE-UP; PLACE CARBON FACE-DOWN ON PHOTO; PLACE PATTERN ON TOP- FACE-UP.

TAPE EDGES

4. FIRMLY TRACE THE PATTERN WITH A BALL POINT PEN.

5. CUT OUT THE PUZZLE PIECES AND PACKAGE IT IN A DECORATIVE ENVELOPE.

PATTERNS FOR PUZZLES

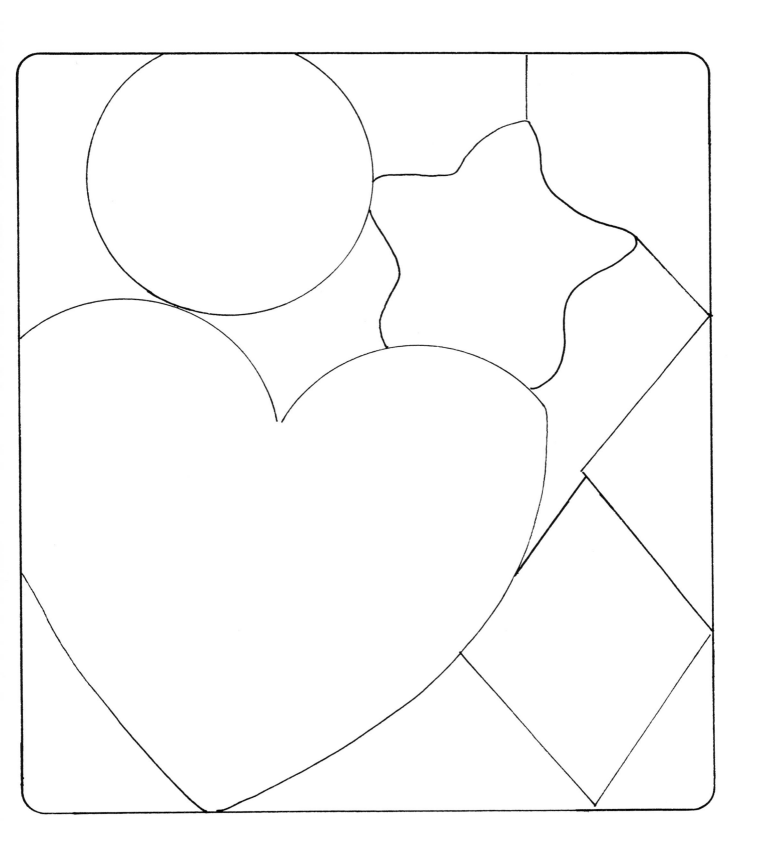

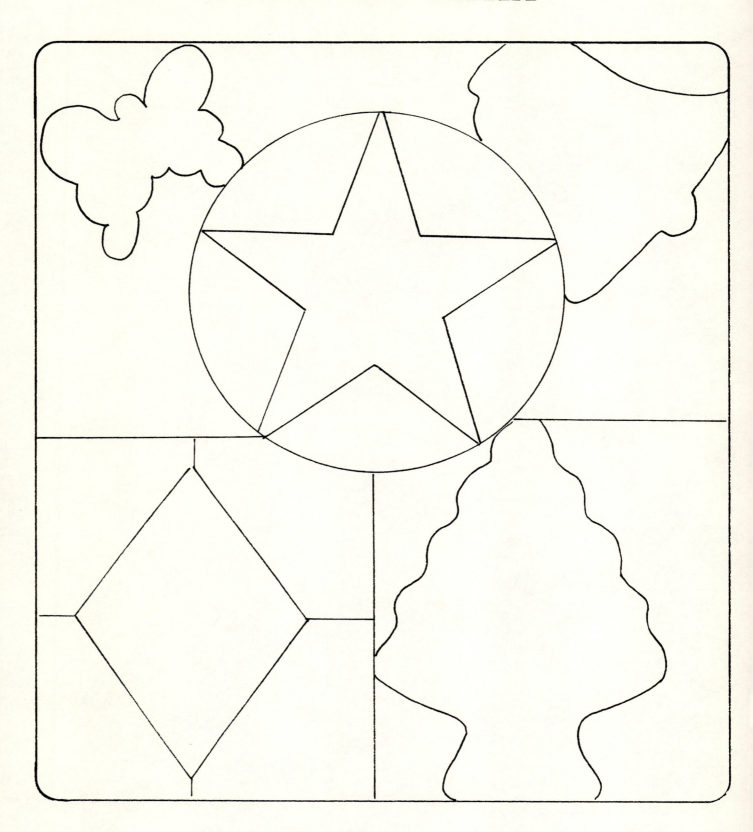

PHOTO COLLAGE

Level of difficulty: *-*****

MATERIALS: White or colored poster board, colored construction paper, glue stick or roll-on paper glue, straight or decorative edging scissors, family pictures, and magazines.

APPLICATIONS: Young people can give these collages to friends and family members for special occasions, while seniors can give them as a pictorial record of their family's heritage.

PREPARATION BEFORE CRAFT SESSION: Collect photographs. Have a quick copy facility economically copy the photos in black and white or color. (You can now return the original photographs.) Cut out construction paper in various shapes and colors; for example, hearts, stars, circles, ovals, and rectangles. Cut out magazine pictures to enhance the photographs or to use in lieu of photographs for those who could not supply their own family photos. These magazine pictures can be of pets, vacations, careers, locales, and miscellaneous family activities.

CRAFT SESSION: Glue the photos on the construction cut-outs; arrange these with magazine pictures (if desired) on the poster board. Secure them with glue. Some participants may wish to further personalize the collages with messages, dates, signatures, etc. You may want to take the finished collages back to the quick copy facility to make multiple copies for gifts.

PHOTO COLLAGE

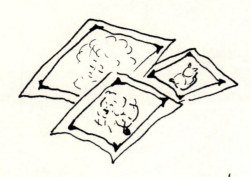

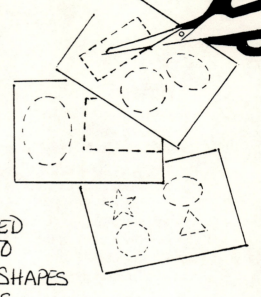

1. COLLECT PHOTOS & MAKE COPIES.

2. CUT COLORED PAPER INTO VARIOUS SHAPES AND SIZES.

3. CUT OUT MAGAZINE PICTURES TO ENHANCE THE COLLAGES.

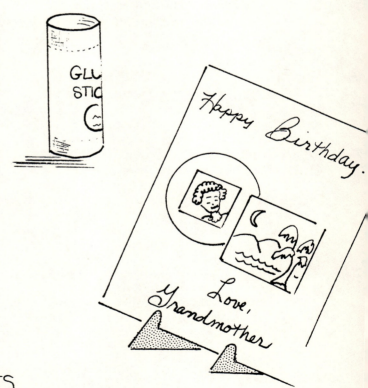

Happy Birthday.

Love, Grandmother

4. GLUE PHOTOS ON THE CUT-OUTS & ARRANGE ON POSTER BOARDS.

5. ADD PERSONAL MESSAGES AND SIGNATURES.

102

PHOTO COLLAGE PATTERNS

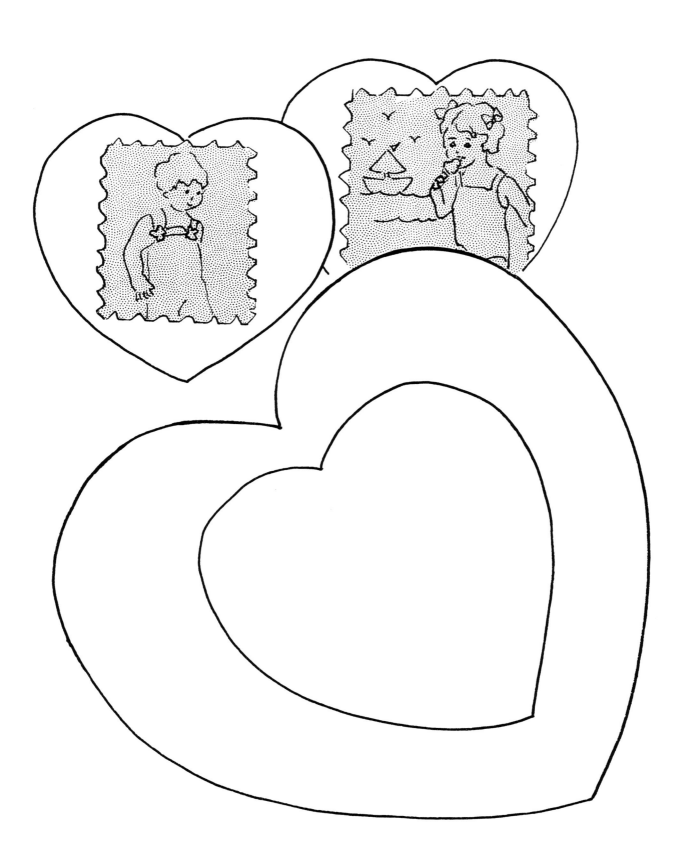

PHOTO COLLAGE PATTERNS

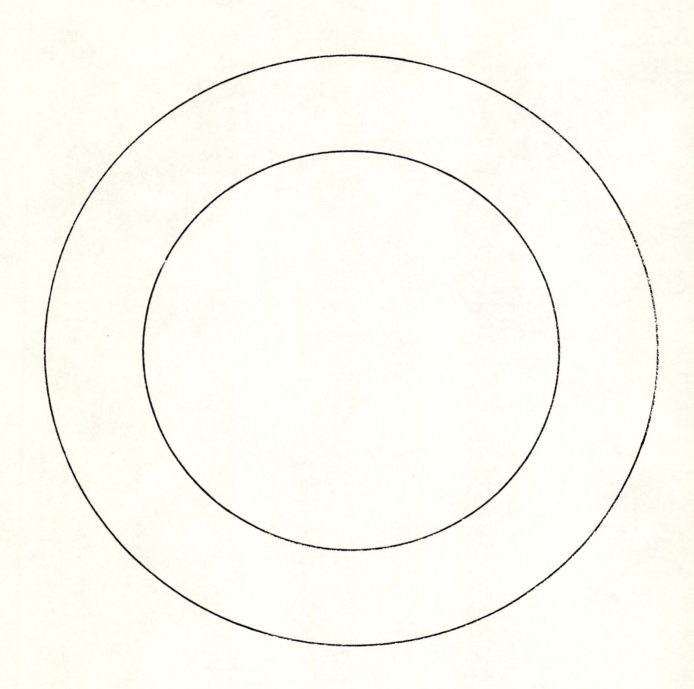

PHOTO COLLAGE PATTERNS

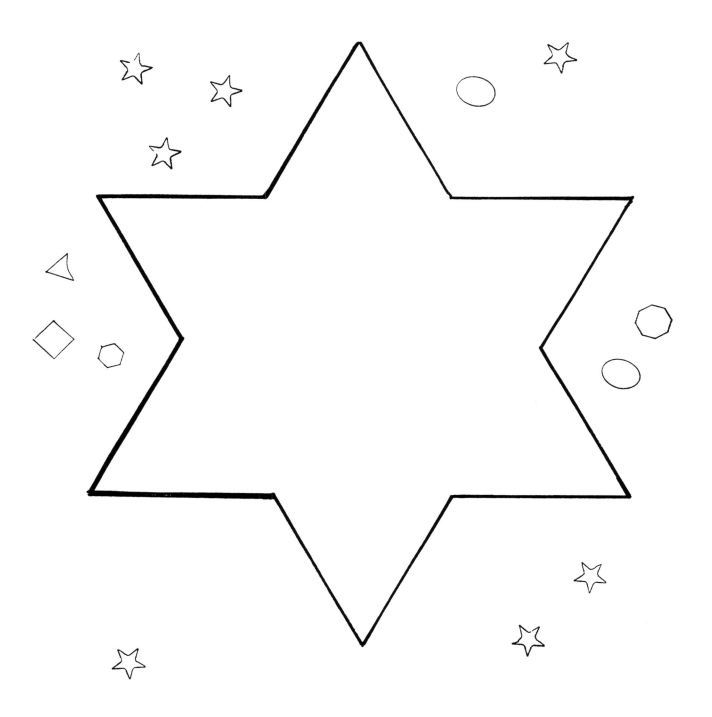

PHOTO COLLAGE PATTERNS

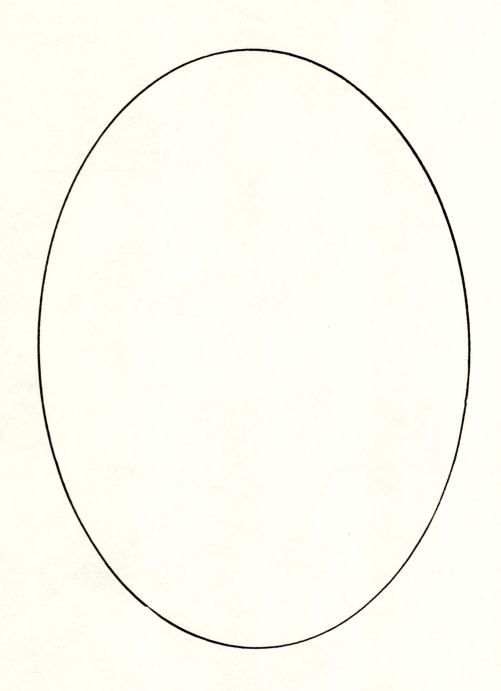

AUTOBIOGRAPHY

Level of difficulty: ***-*****

MATERIALS: Tape recorders, lined and unlined paper, pens and pencils, drawing materials, construction paper, paper punch or stapler, yarn or brads, $9 \times 12''$ envelopes.

APPLICATIONS: Autobiographies make great gifts or favors for family reunions and holiday dinners.

PREPARATION BEFORE CRAFT SESSION: Arrange a transcriber, family or volunteer, for each participant. Have a training session for the transcribers. Give them a list of facilitating questions and topics. For example, you may want to ask about family traditions for birthdays and holidays, vacations, memorable picnics, senior proms, first kiss, first love, first car, hobbies, pets, children, careers.

CRAFT SESSION: Introduce the concept of autobiographies. They can be retrospective accounts of special incidents for one session, or more detailed biographies for multiple sessions. Introduce the transcribers. Store the tapes and notes in $9 \times 12''$ envelopes between sessions. Be sure to put names on the envelopes. You may want to have an additional session to illustrate the notes or to design a cover. See Decorative Boxes in this book for ideas to attractively package the tapes for gifts. You can assemble a cover for notes with a construction paper cover.

AUTOBIOGRAPHY

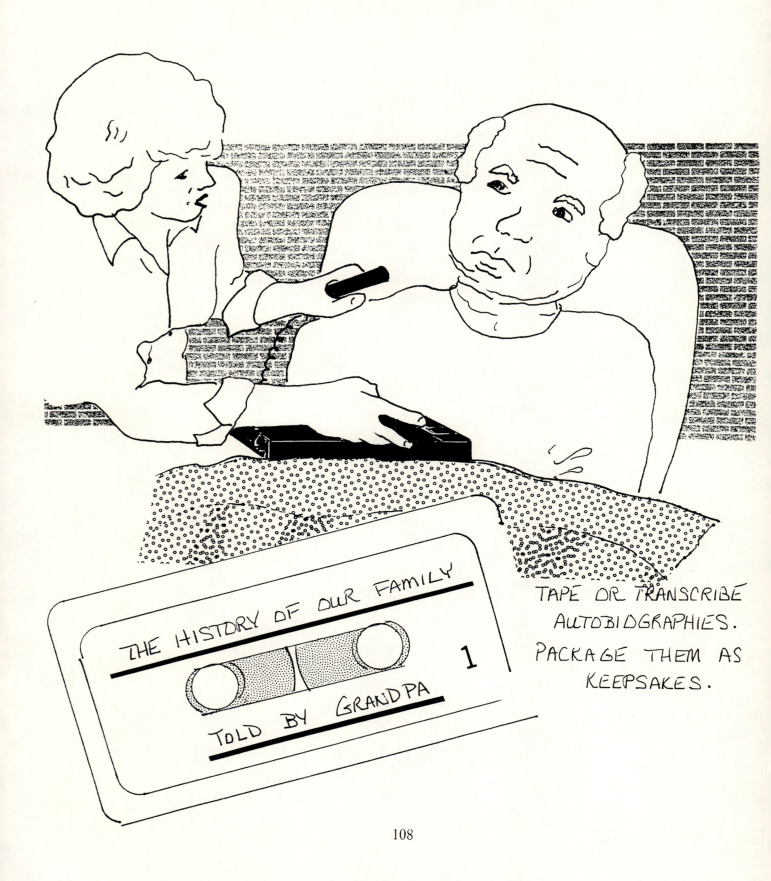

THE HISTORY OF OUR FAMILY

TOLD BY GRANDPA

1

TAPE OR TRANSCRIBE AUTOBIOGRAPHIES. PACKAGE THEM AS KEEPSAKES.

SOUP RECIPES

Level of difficulty: **-*****

MATERIALS: Empty soup can with label, plastic vegetables or flowers, floral clay or Styrofoam, plastic fork, 5 × 7 file card, recipes, black felt marking pens.

APPLICATIONS: Most people have a favorite recipe to share with their families. This is a pretty reminder of "Aunt Esther's" wisdom and also makes a unique and special kitchen shower gift.

PREPARATION BEFORE CRAFT SESSION: Wash soup cans carefully taking care not to soil the label, which remains on the can. Bring a recipe for each type soup can you have for those people who cannot remember or do not have their own recipes (example: Split pea, vegetable, onion, chicken).

CRAFT SESSION: Fill the can with clay or Styrofoam. Using the plastic vegetables and flowers, make an attractive arrangement with the can as the vase. Insert a plastic fork upside down into the arrangement. Help each person write down his favorite recipe on a file card. Be sure to include signatures or names. Then insert the card through the tines of the fork.

SOUP RECIPES

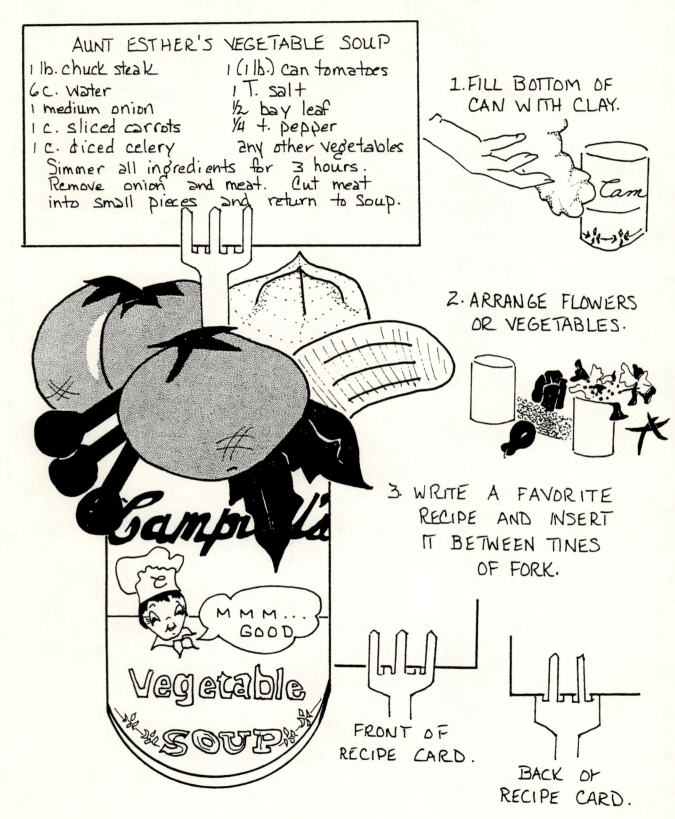

AUNT ESTHER'S VEGETABLE SOUP

1 lb. chuck steak	1 (1 lb.) can tomatoes
6 c. water	1 T. salt
1 medium onion	½ bay leaf
1 c. sliced carrots	¼ t. pepper
1 c. diced celery	any other vegetables

Simmer all ingredients for 3 hours. Remove onion and meat. Cut meat into small pieces and return to soup.

1. FILL BOTTOM OF CAN WITH CLAY.

2. ARRANGE FLOWERS OR VEGETABLES.

3. WRITE A FAVORITE RECIPE AND INSERT IT BETWEEN TINES OF FORK.

FRONT OF RECIPE CARD.

BACK OF RECIPE CARD.

EXTRA RECIPES

SPLIT PEA SOUP

1 large ham bone
1 lb. split peas
3 quarts water
1 white onion
1/2 carrot (diced)

Salt, red & white pepper
6 slices bacon (optional)
2 hard cooked eggs
(optional)

Boil peas and ham until peas dissolve. Add seasoning and simmer 2½ hours. Put soup through sieve. Replace ham bits in soup. Sprinkle bacon crumbs & chopped egg over each serving.

TOMATO SOUP

2 c. tomato juice
1 rib celery
1/4 medium green pepper
2 medium carrots
1 medium tomato
1/2 cucumber

salt
tobasco
pepper
worcestershire sauce
1/2 sliced lime or lemon

Chop all vegetables. Add seasoning to taste. Chill thoroughly. Serve in bowl with slice of lime.

CHICKEN SOUP

3 lb. hen
3 quarts water
3 c. chopped celery
1 large onion
2 carrots, diced

6 sprigs parsley
1/4 t. thyme
1 T. salt
1/4 t. pepper

Simmer all ingredients 3 hours. Pour through a sieve. Save chicken for salads. Rice or noodles may then be cooked in the broth.

LUNCH BAGS

Level of difficulty: *-**

MATERIALS: Colored art paper, lunch bags, scissors, craft glue, brush.

APPLICATIONS: Children adore decorated lunch bags for school or camp. Patients can even personalize the bags with their grandchildren's names worked into the design. These bags are almost too easy to make, but they are clever and eye-catching. They are just the project to interest an otherwise reluctant person. We especially like to cut out the designs nonchalantly while carrying on conversations with our patients. They became intrigued and were more open to mutual participation in a project the next time they were asked. These bags can be adapted to be used as gift bags.

PREPARATION BEFORE CRAFT SESSION: Cut designs out of colored paper. Curl eyelashes, whiskers, and hair by winding the paper tightly around the end of a brush and then releasing it. Be creative or copy the patterns in the illustrations.

CRAFT SESSION: Apply glue to the cutouts. Press in place. Cut out names and "lunch" or "bag" out of paper, and glue these on too.

LUNCH BAGS

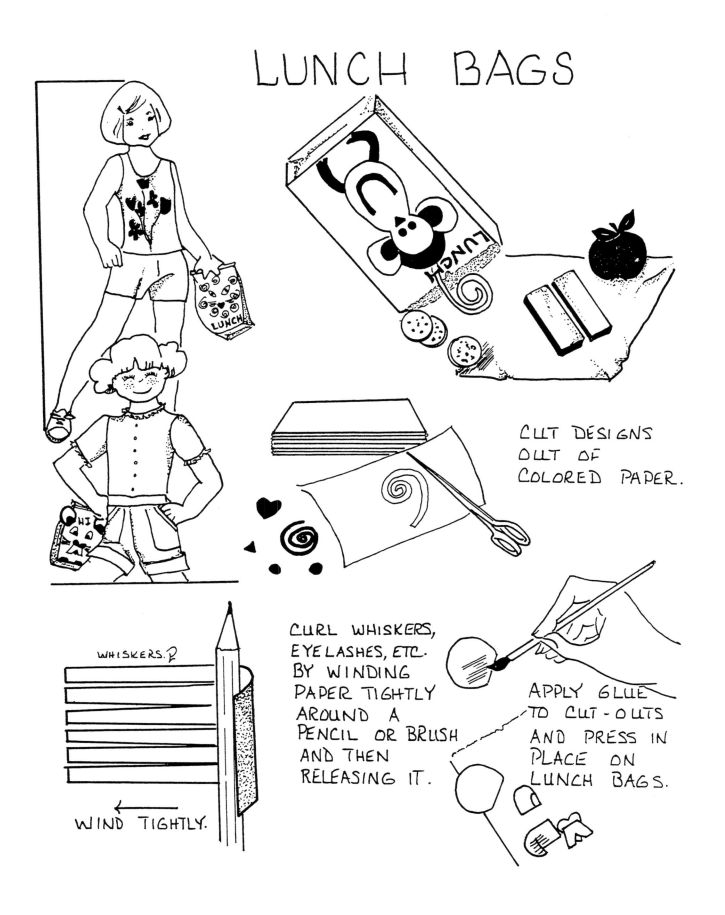

CUT DESIGNS OUT OF COLORED PAPER.

CURL WHISKERS, EYELASHES, ETC. BY WINDING PAPER TIGHTLY AROUND A PENCIL OR BRUSH AND THEN RELEASING IT.

APPLY GLUE TO CUT-OUTS AND PRESS IN PLACE ON LUNCH BAGS.

WHISKERS.

WIND TIGHTLY.

113

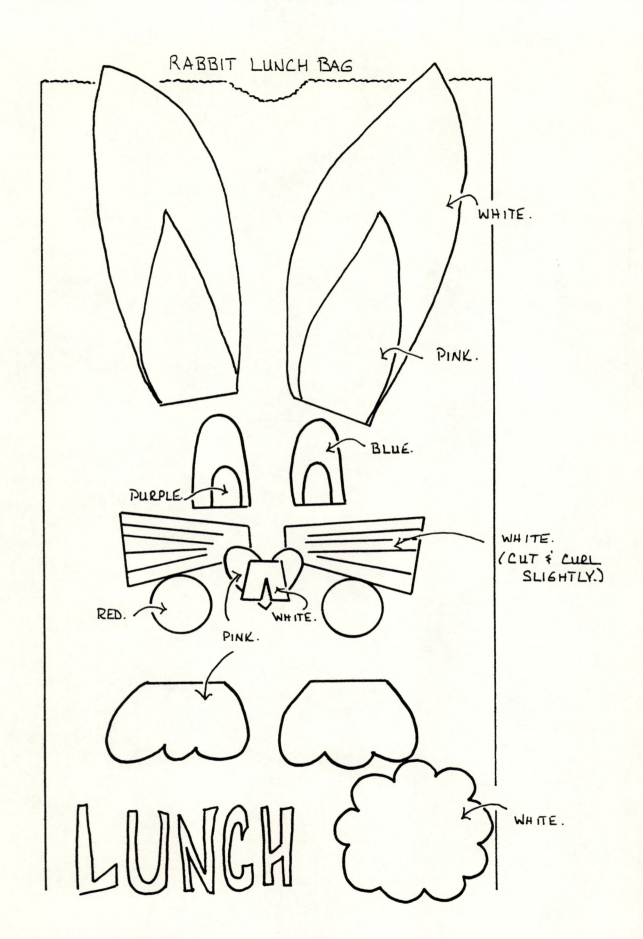

RABBIT LUNCH BAG

WHITE.

PINK.

BLUE.

PURPLE.

WHITE.
(CUT & CURL
SLIGHTLY.)

RED.

WHITE.

PINK.

WHITE.

LUNCH

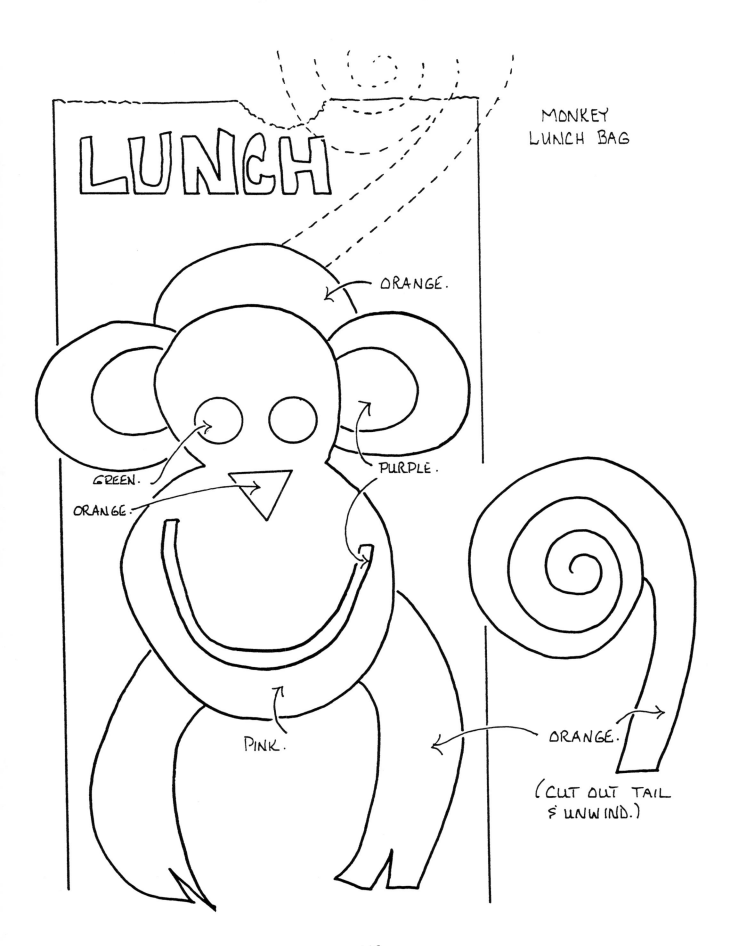

MONKEY
LUNCH BAG

LUNCH

ORANGE.

GREEN.

ORANGE.

PURPLE.

PINK.

ORANGE.

(CUT OUT TAIL
& UNWIND.)

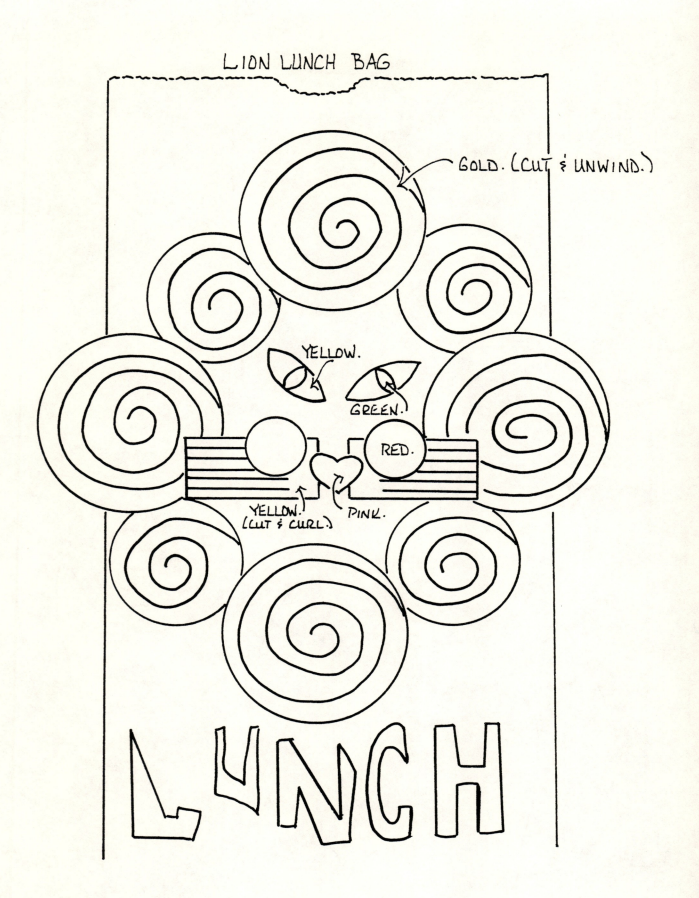

RED RIDING HOOD LUNCH BAG

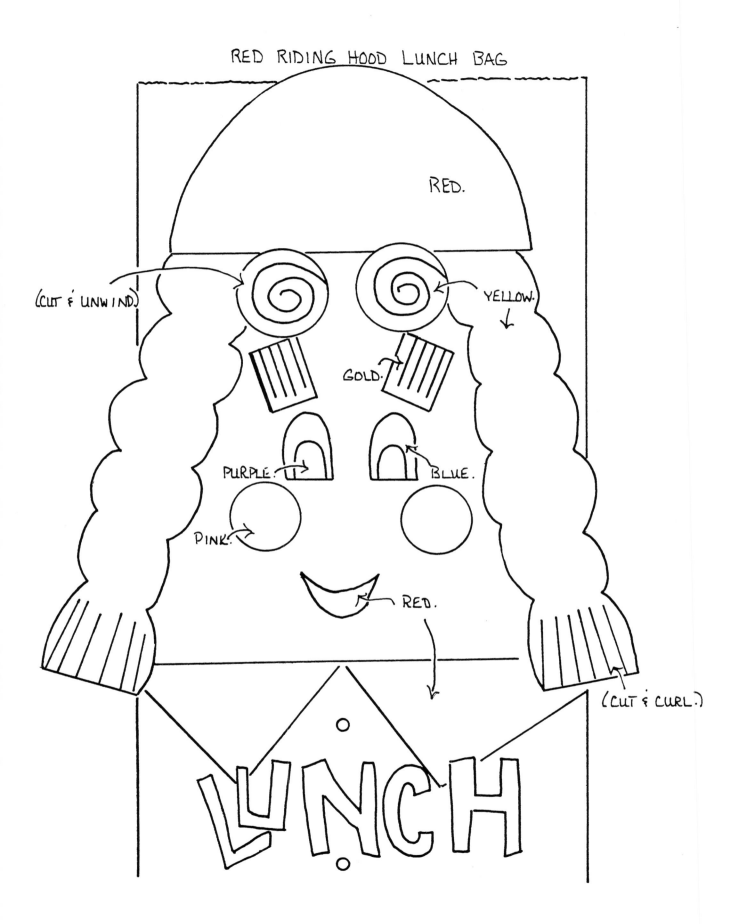

CAT LUNCH BAG

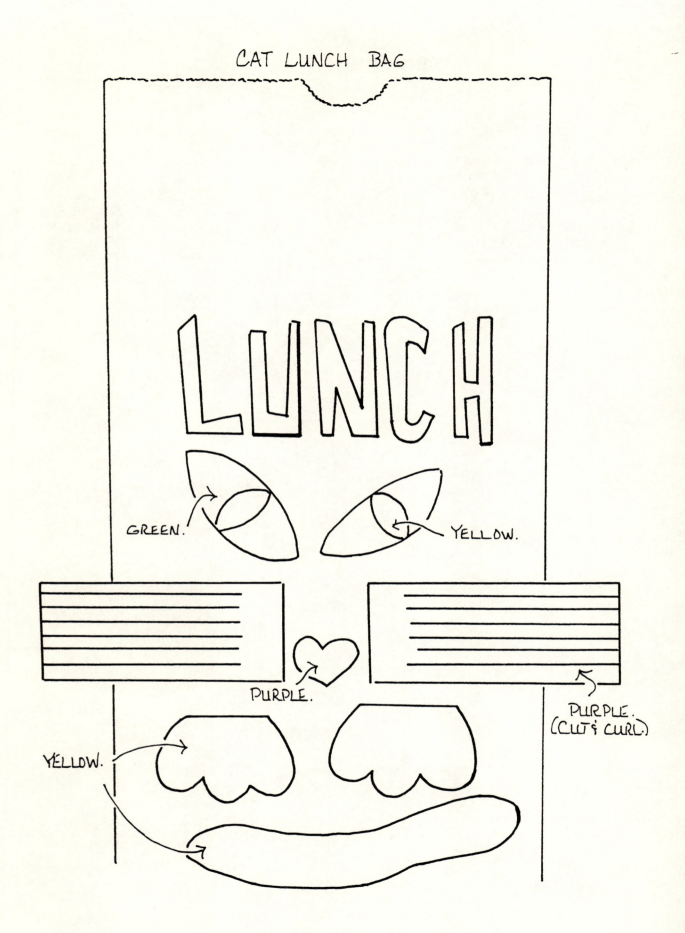

118

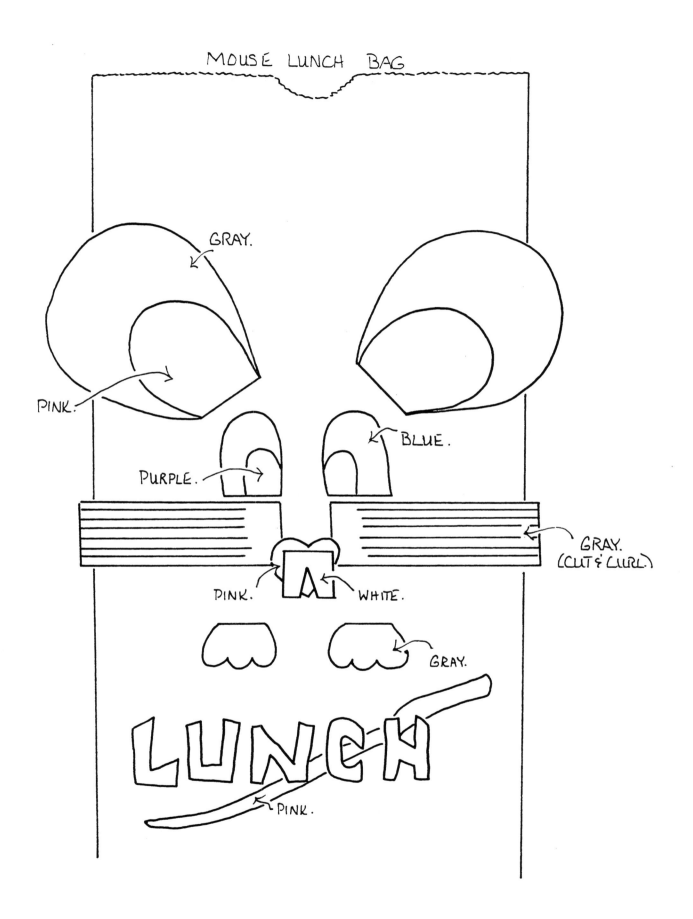

MOUSE LUNCH BAG

GRAY.

PINK.

BLUE.

PURPLE.

GRAY.
(CUT & CURL.)

PINK. WHITE.

GRAY.

LUNCH

PINK.

119

CANDY BOWL

Level of difficulty: *-**

MATERIALS: Empty margarine tubs, 27 round-headed clothespins for each bowl, wood stain (optional).

APPLICATIONS: It is hard to believe this candy bowl was once a margarine tub and clothespins. Fill it with mints before giving it away for an extra nice gift.

PREPARATION BEFORE CRAFT SESSION: If you like, stain the clothespins and allow them to dry.

CRAFT SESSION: Simply put the clothespins over the edge of the tub and push them close together. Fill the bowl with candy for a clothespin studded candy bowl.

CANDY BOWL

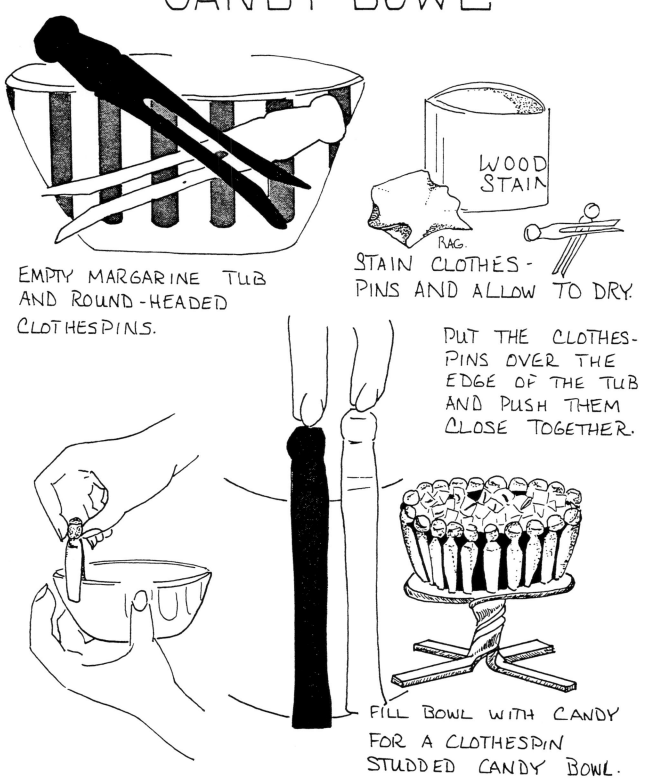

EMPTY MARGARINE TUB
AND ROUND-HEADED
CLOTHESPINS.

WOOD
STAIN

RAG.

STAIN CLOTHES-
PINS AND ALLOW TO DRY.

PUT THE CLOTHES-
PINS OVER THE
EDGE OF THE TUB
AND PUSH THEM
CLOSE TOGETHER.

FILL BOWL WITH CANDY
FOR A CLOTHESPIN
STUDDED CANDY BOWL.

LOLLIPOP BASKETS

Level of difficulty: **-***

MATERIALS: Empty plastic produce baskets, ribbon, 1-inch thick Styrofoam, lollipops, knife.

APPLICATIONS: A whole basket of lollipops appeals to every child. If you do not have a special child in mind for your basket, donate it to a local hospital.

PREPARATION BEFORE CRAFT SESSION: Cut the Styrofoam in squares to exactly fit the bottom of a basket.

CRAFT SESSION: Weave ribbon around the basket and tie it in a bow. Put a piece of Styrofoam in the bottom of the basket. Poke the lollipops into the Styrofoam. Be sure no one with diabetes eats a lollipop.

LOLLIPOP BASKETS

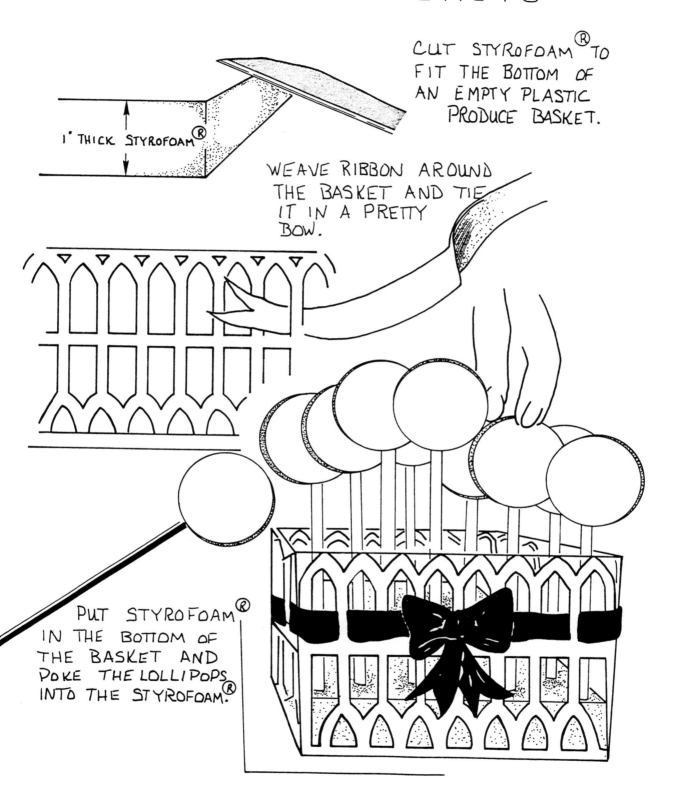

CUT STYROFOAM® TO FIT THE BOTTOM OF AN EMPTY PLASTIC PRODUCE BASKET.

1" THICK STYROFOAM®

WEAVE RIBBON AROUND THE BASKET AND TIE IT IN A PRETTY BOW.

PUT STYROFOAM® IN THE BOTTOM OF THE BASKET AND POKE THE LOLLIPOPS INTO THE STYROFOAM®.

TOY SNAKES

Level of difficulty: ***-*****

MATERIALS: Fabric, toilet paper tubes, buttons, red ribbon or bias binding, knee socks or stockings, paper towels, glue, pinking shears (stapler and staples optional).

APPLICATIONS: The wiggly toy snakes appeal to young grandchildren. They also make a nice contribution to a local church or school bazaar or the pediatric ward of a hospital.

PREPARATION BEFORE CRAFT SESSION: Cut red forked tongues about 3 inches in length. Cut fabric (calico is especially appealing) into pieces 5 inches by 6 inches.

CRAFT SESSION: Cover five tubes with cloth for each snake. The simplest way is to paint a stripe of glue down a tube. Secure the cloth. Then wind the cloth around the tube and glue the overlap. Stuff paper towels into the toe of a sock to form the head. String the tubes onto the sock, knotting several socks together for added length. When the last one is on, tie a large knot in the tail end. Then glue on two buttons for the eyes and the ribbon for the tongue. The end knot may be stapled to the end tube for added security. Be cautious that buttons are not swallowed.

TOY SNAKES

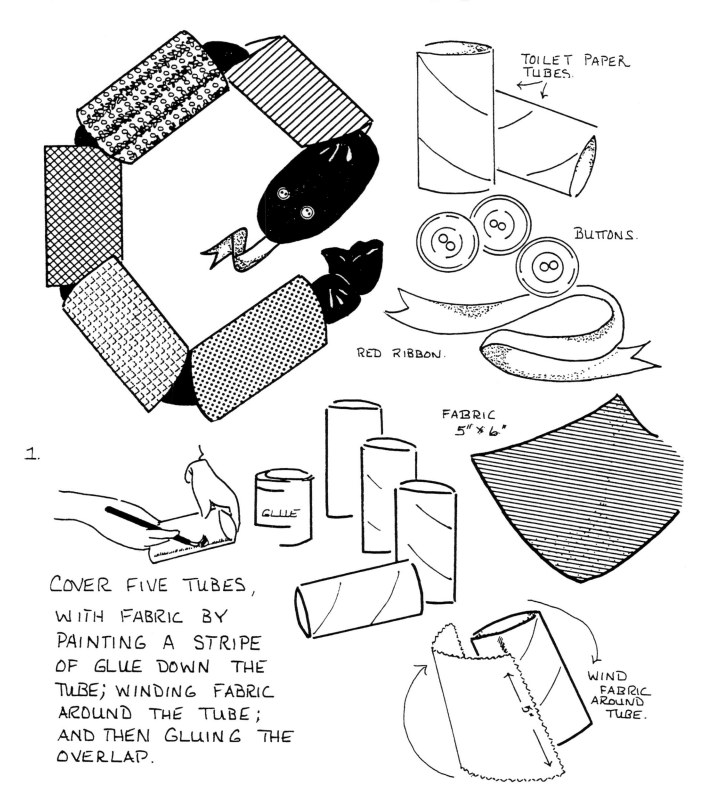

TOILET PAPER TUBES.

BUTTONS.

RED RIBBON.

FABRIC 5" × 6"

GLUE

1. COVER FIVE TUBES, WITH FABRIC BY PAINTING A STRIPE OF GLUE DOWN THE TUBE; WINDING FABRIC AROUND THE TUBE; AND THEN GLUING THE OVERLAP.

WIND FABRIC AROUND TUBE.

5"

TOY SNAKES

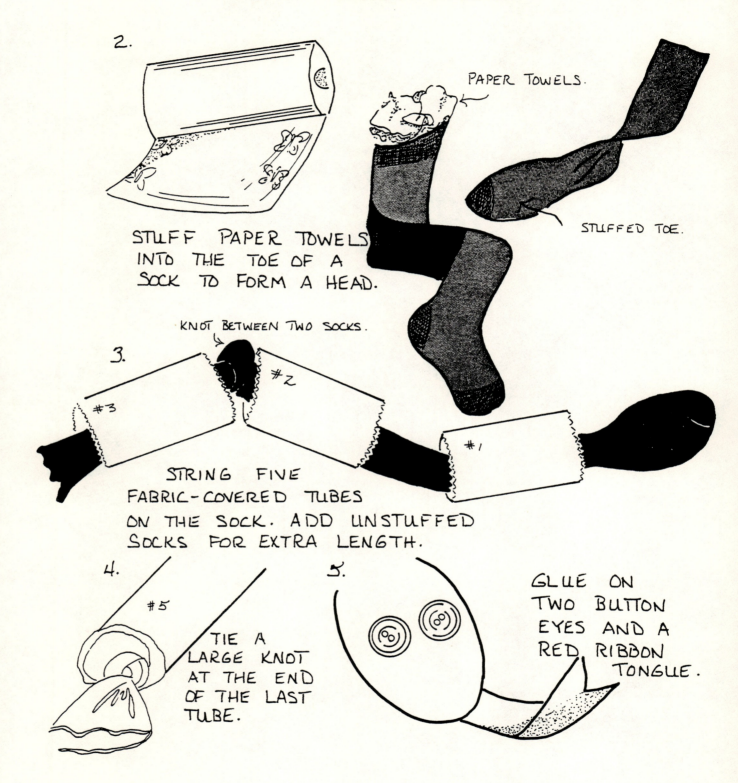

2.

PAPER TOWELS.

STUFFED TOE.

STUFF PAPER TOWELS INTO THE TOE OF A SOCK TO FORM A HEAD.

KNOT BETWEEN TWO SOCKS.

3.

#3

#2

#1

STRING FIVE FABRIC-COVERED TUBES ON THE SOCK. ADD UNSTUFFED SOCKS FOR EXTRA LENGTH.

4.

#5

TIE A LARGE KNOT AT THE END OF THE LAST TUBE.

5.

GLUE ON TWO BUTTON EYES AND A RED RIBBON TONGUE.

126

PATTERNS FOR TOY SNAKE

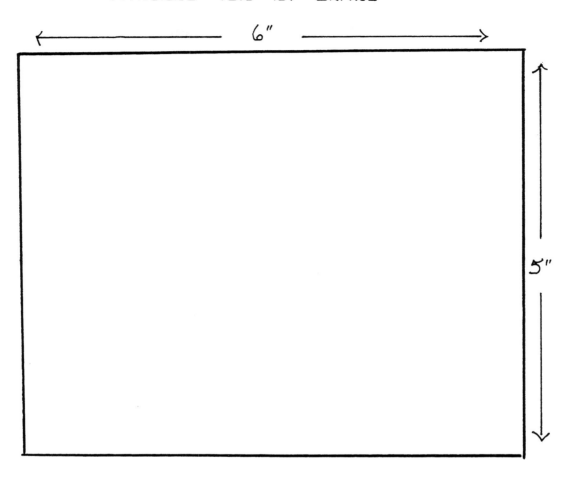

USE PINKING SHEARS TO CUT FIVE
PIECES OF FABRIC FOR EACH SNAKE.

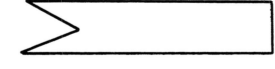

CUT ONE TONGUE PER SNAKE.

EASTER EGGS

Level of difficulty: *-*****

MATERIALS: Eggs, needle, felt marking pens in a variety of colors, empty egg cartons, cellophane grass, paper bowls or baskets of any sort (example: empty plastic produce baskets).

APPLICATIONS: Personalized Easter eggs are special to family members; and if stored carefully, they stay pretty for years to display annually.

PREPARATION BEFORE CRAFT SESSION: Separate each egg section from a carton to serve as egg-holders for feeble hands that might otherwise crack a blown egg. Then blow eggs. To do this, begin by shaking the egg. Use a needle to make a hole at one end of the egg and another one a bit larger at the other end. Blow gently into the smaller hole until the yolk and white are completely out. Wash the shell and stand it on end to dry. (You can use the eggs for baking.) Note that a large rubber syringe can be used to blow out the egg, if you prefer a tool.

CRAFT SESSION: Put a blown egg in an egg carton section and let each person decorate in their own creative ways. Traditional Easter bunnies and flowers are nice, but so are zig zags and colorful scribbling. Assemble half a dozen eggs on the cellophane grass in bowls or baskets.

EASTER EGGS

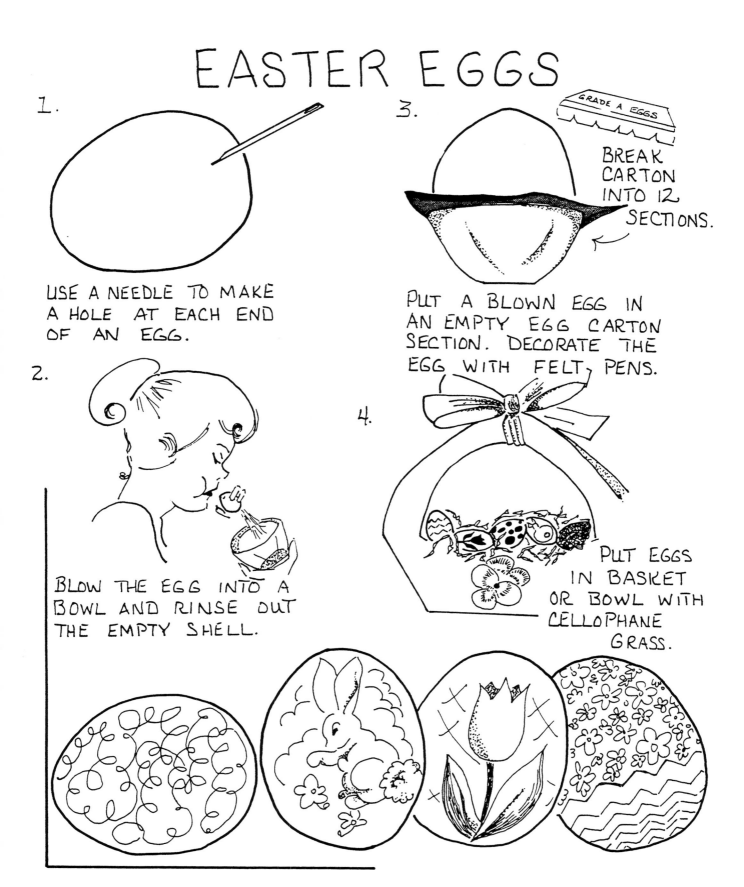

1.

USE A NEEDLE TO MAKE A HOLE AT EACH END OF AN EGG.

2.

BLOW THE EGG INTO A BOWL AND RINSE OUT THE EMPTY SHELL.

3.

GRADE A EGGS

BREAK CARTON INTO 12 SECTIONS.

PUT A BLOWN EGG IN AN EMPTY EGG CARTON SECTION. DECORATE THE EGG WITH FELT PENS.

4.

PUT EGGS IN BASKET OR BOWL WITH CELLOPHANE GRASS.

SAVINGS BANKS

Level of difficulty: *-***

MATERIALS: Empty pop-top soda cans, plain art paper, glue stick, craft glue, black felt marking pen, crayons, scissors, ric rac or ribbon, small paint brush, gummed labels (3 inch × 3 inch).

APPLICATIONS: Grandchildren especially like personalized little banks with their names on the outside and a couple of pennies that jingle on the inside. The banks are also nice to save a few coins for your favorite charity.

PREPARATION BEFORE CRAFT SESSION: Cut plain art paper to fit around pop-top soda cans (4½ inch × 8¼ inch). Trace patterns on the paper with a black felt pen. Using glue stick, secure the paper to the table in front of each person.

CRAFT SESSION: Have each person color the patterns with crayon. Using a paint brush, spread craft glue on the can and attach the colored pattern. Glue a trim of ric rac or ribbon on the top and bottom of the can. Then help each person design and write a personalized label for the can. Be sure to include a signature. Attach the label to the can.

SAVINGS BANKS

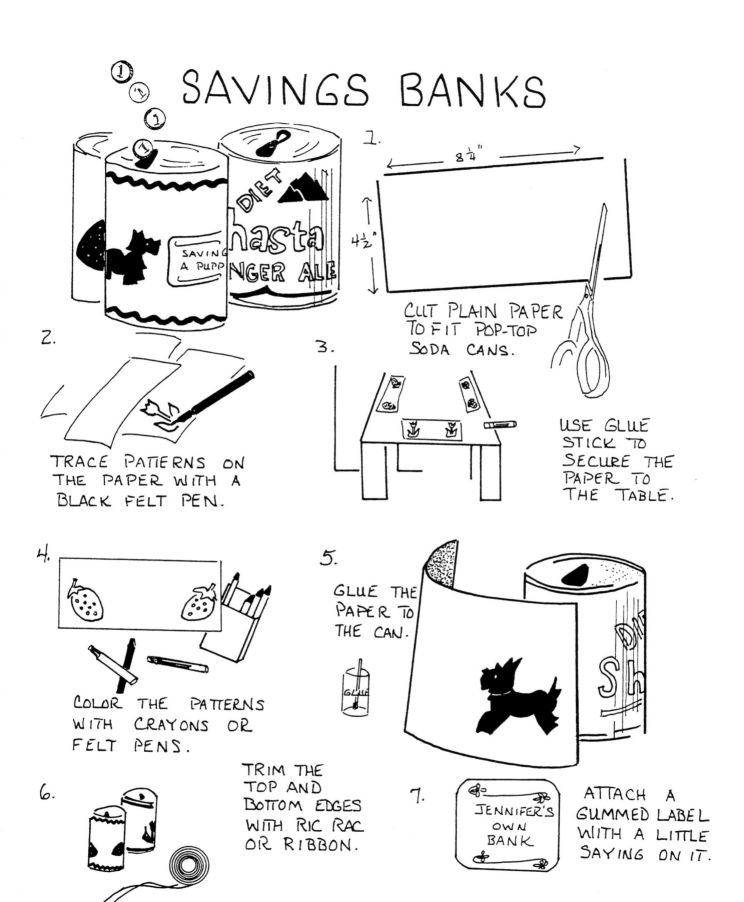

1. CUT PLAIN PAPER TO FIT POP-TOP SODA CANS.

8¼"

4½"

2. TRACE PATTERNS ON THE PAPER WITH A BLACK FELT PEN.

3. USE GLUE STICK TO SECURE THE PAPER TO THE TABLE.

4. COLOR THE PATTERNS WITH CRAYONS OR FELT PENS.

5. GLUE THE PAPER TO THE CAN.

6. TRIM THE TOP AND BOTTOM EDGES WITH RIC RAC OR RIBBON.

7. ATTACH A GUMMED LABEL WITH A LITTLE SAYING ON IT.

JENNIFER'S OWN BANK

PATTERNS FOR SAVINGS BANKS

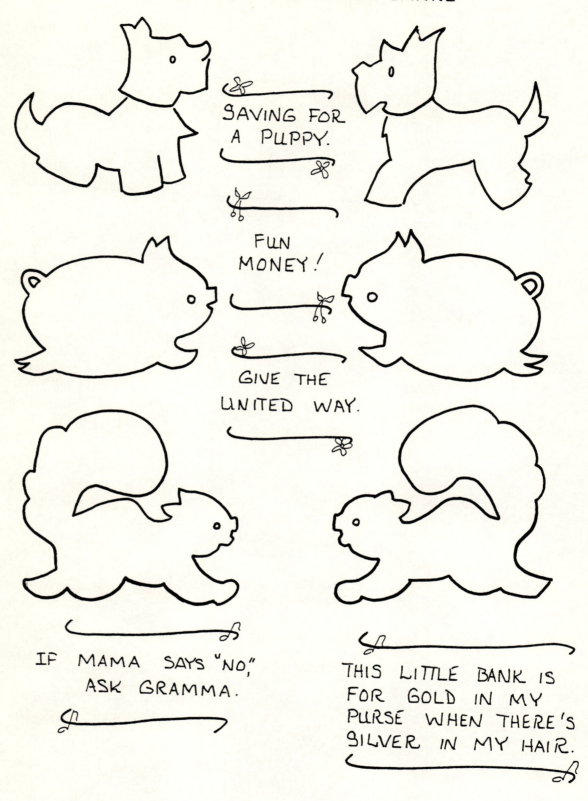

SAVING FOR A PUPPY.

FUN MONEY!

GIVE THE UNITED WAY.

IF MAMA SAYS "NO," ASK GRAMMA.

THIS LITTLE BANK IS FOR GOLD IN MY PURSE WHEN THERE'S SILVER IN MY HAIR.

CANDY CLOWN

Level of difficulty: *****

MATERIALS: Cardboard, fabric scraps, 2½ inch plastic flower pots, empty baby food jars, empty medicine cups, ball trim or cotton balls, ric rac (optional), colored paper (red, pink, blue, purple, yellow), craft glue, brush, scissors, pinking shears, candy and gum.

APPLICATIONS: Candy clowns are sure to bring smiles to children's faces. Seniors can give them to their grandchildren, and children can give them to their friends. The clowns are made from items usually thrown away. The baby food jars are easily found in hospital or nursing home kitchens. Patients especially like to save their medicine cups for craft projects. And nurseries are always glad to give away their used plastic pots. Just ask for them.

PREPARATION BEFORE CRAFT SESSION: Using the cardboard, cut one hat base and one foot base for each clown. Then with the pinking shears and fabric, cut five collars, one hat, one hat base, and one foot base for each clown. Cut out eyes, hair, cheeks, and lips from the colored paper or felt.

CRAFT SESSION: Glue the fabric to the cardboard foot base and hat base. Trim the feet with ric rac and ball trim or cotton balls. Glue the five cloth collars to the outside lip of the jar. Glue the jar onto the foot base, fill the jar with candy and gum. Turn the flower pot upside down and glue on the face and hair. Glue the fabric hat around the medicine cup, which has also been turned upside down. Then glue the hat to the hat base and then the completed hat to the bottom of the flower pot. Attach a ball trim or cotton ball to the tip of the hat, and put the clown face lid on the candy-filled jar.

CANDY CLOWN

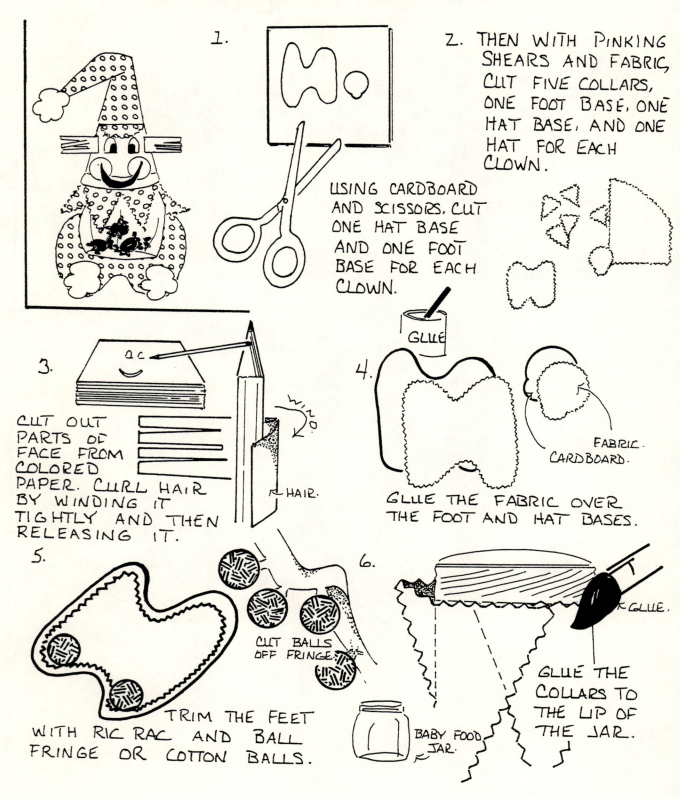

1.

2. THEN WITH PINKING SHEARS AND FABRIC, CUT FIVE COLLARS, ONE FOOT BASE, ONE HAT BASE, AND ONE HAT FOR EACH CLOWN.

USING CARDBOARD AND SCISSORS, CUT ONE HAT BASE AND ONE FOOT BASE FOR EACH CLOWN.

GLUE

3. CUT OUT PARTS OF FACE FROM COLORED PAPER. CURL HAIR BY WINDING IT TIGHTLY AND THEN RELEASING IT.

WIND

HAIR.

4. FABRIC. CARDBOARD.

GLUE THE FABRIC OVER THE FOOT AND HAT BASES.

5. TRIM THE FEET WITH RIC RAC AND BALL FRINGE OR COTTON BALLS.

CUT BALLS OFF FRINGE.

6. GLUE.

GLUE THE COLLARS TO THE LIP OF THE JAR.

BABY FOOD JAR.

CANDY CLOWN

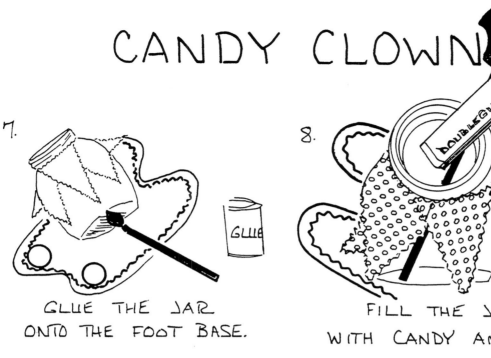

7.

GLUE THE JAR
ONTO THE FOOT BASE.

8.

FILL THE JAR
WITH CANDY AND GUM.

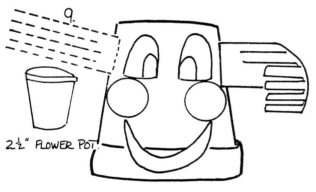

9.

2½" FLOWER POT.

TURN FLOWER POT UPSIDE
DOWN AND GLUE ON FACE.

10.

CONE. →

WRAP FABRIC
HAT AROUND
UPSIDE DOWN
MEDICINE CUP
AND GLUE IT
TO FORM A
CONE.

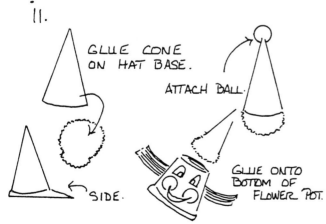

11.

GLUE CONE
ON HAT BASE.

ATTACH BALL.

GLUE ONTO
BOTTOM OF
FLOWER POT.

← SIDE.

FINISH THE HAT.

12.

PUT CLOWN FACE "LID"
ON CANDY FILLED JAR.

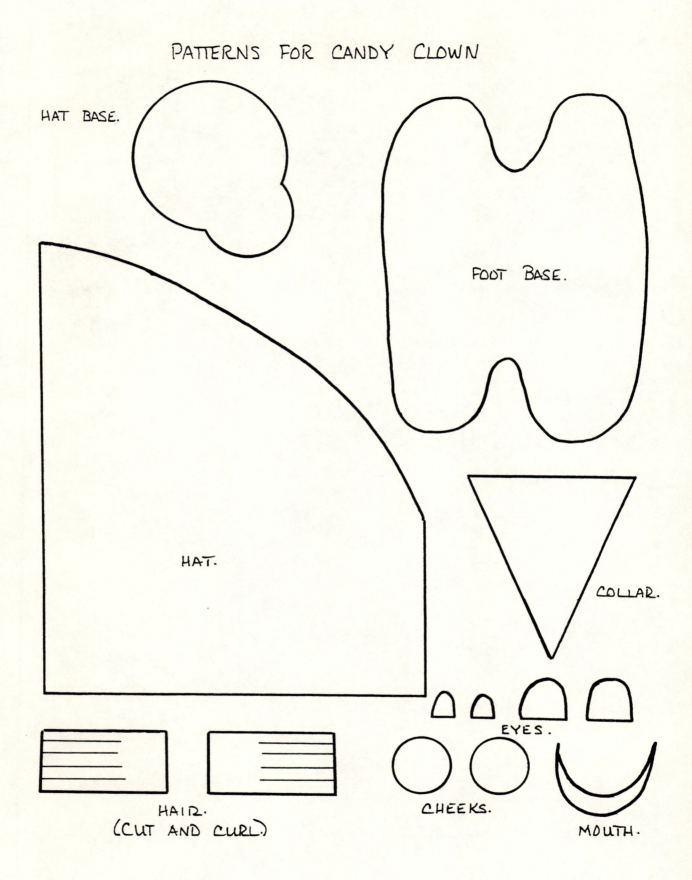

PATTERNS FOR CANDY CLOWN

HAT BASE.

FOOT BASE.

HAT.

COLLAR.

EYES.

HAIR.
(CUT AND CURL.)

CHEEKS.

MOUTH.

BUTTON-ON DOGGIES

Level of difficulty: ***-****

MATERIALS: Scissors, buttons, needles, thread, single-edged razors, thimble, leatherette samples or heavy oil cloth, adhesive tape, felt marking pen.

APPLICATIONS: These cute *button-on doggies* are used to lengthen shoulder straps on overalls and suspenders. They are useful gifts for young mamas who do not have time to re-sew buttons.

PREPARATION BEFORE CRAFT SESSION: Draw sets of doggies on the leatherette and cut them out. Place adhesive tape on the backs of the doggies as illustrated. Using a razor blade, *slice* a button hole in the head of each doggie. Mark the location for each button.

CRAFT SESSION: Sew buttons on the bottom of each doggie. Make lots of sets.

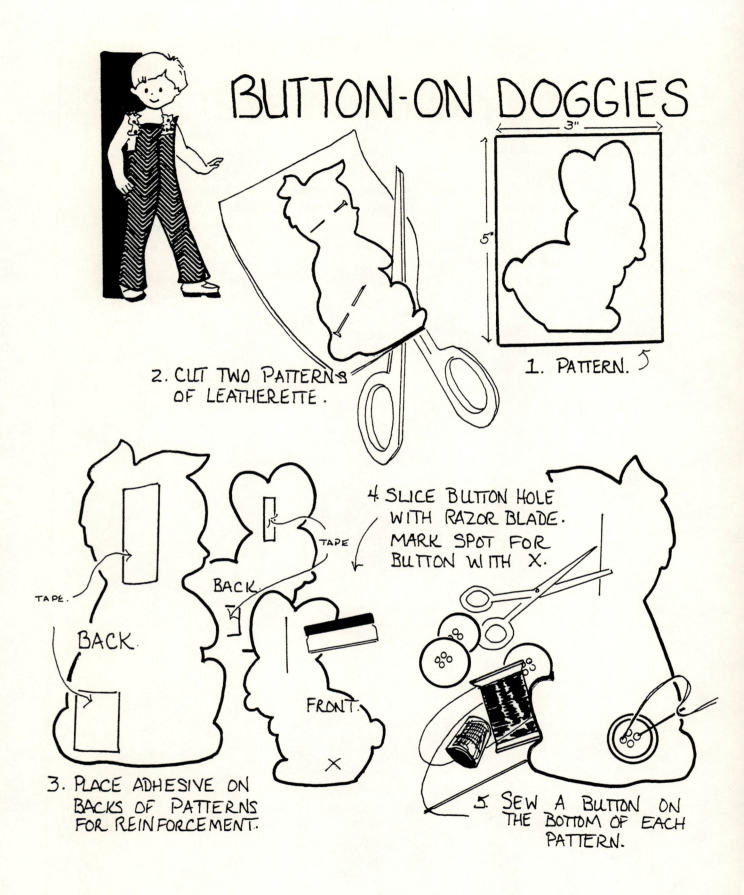

BUTTON-ON DOGGIES

1. PATTERN.

3″

5″

2. CUT TWO PATTERNS OF LEATHERETTE.

3. PLACE ADHESIVE ON BACKS OF PATTERNS FOR REINFORCEMENT.

TAPE.

BACK.

BACK.

TAPE

FRONT.

4. SLICE BUTTON HOLE WITH RAZOR BLADE. MARK SPOT FOR BUTTON WITH X.

5. SEW A BUTTON ON THE BOTTOM OF EACH PATTERN.

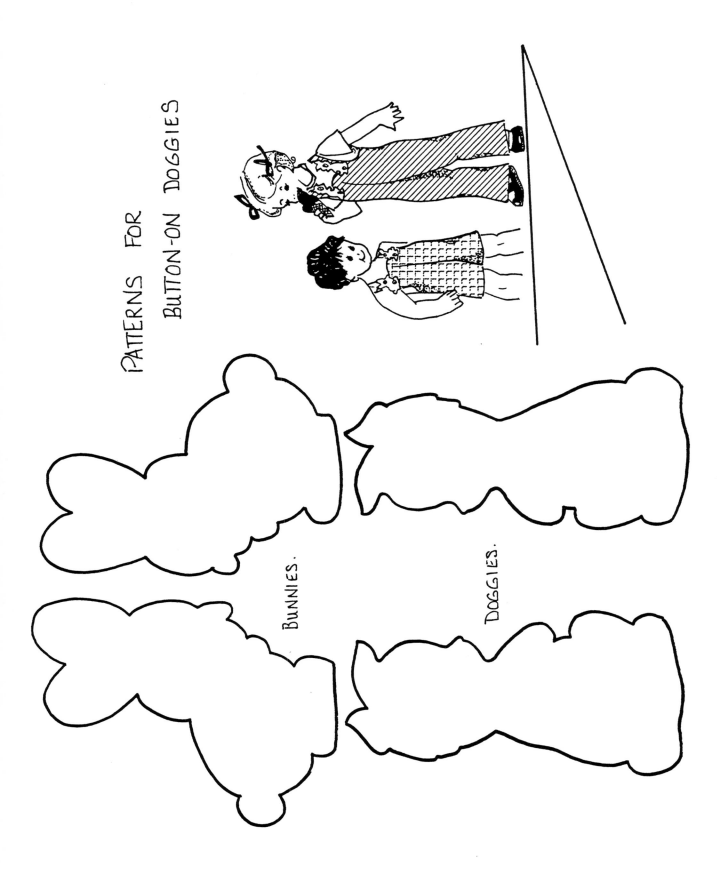

PATTERNS FOR
BUTTON-ON DOGGIES

BUNNIES.

DOGGIES.

139

SHOE TREES

Level of difficulty: *-*****

MATERIALS: Pinking shears, ribbon, old stockings, fabric scraps, (charcoal cedar chips, or potpourri, optional), string or heavy thread, small decorative ornaments (optional).

APPLICATIONS: Every family member will appreciate shoe trees. Make satin ones for ladies and corduroy ones for men, or use pastels and plaids. Tie bows around the ladies'; tie knots around the men's. Note that by stuffing the trees with charcoal, potpourri, or cedar chips, they also become deodorizers.

PREPARATION BEFORE CRAFT SESSION: Cut two matching circles of fabric 14 inches in diameter with a pinking shears for each pair of shoe trees.

CRAFT SESSION: Stuff the toes of the old stockings with fabric scraps and tie with thread. Cover the stuffed stockings with the circles of cloth. Gather the edges together and tie them with ribbon. Pull the edges so that the fabric becomes taut over the stocking. Insert ornaments under the ribbon if desired.

SHOE TREES

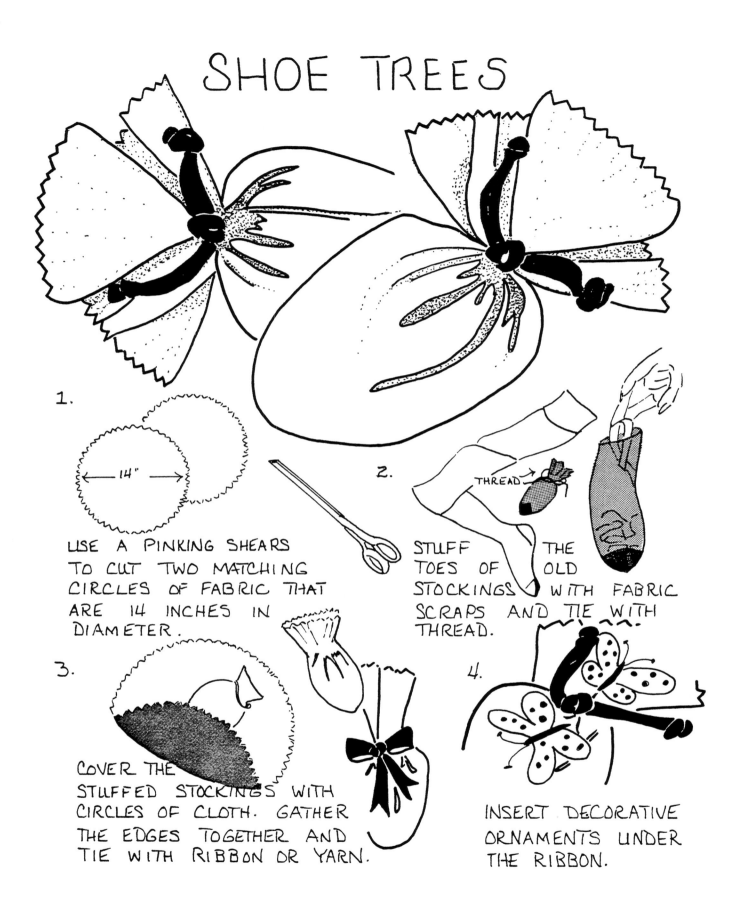

1. USE A PINKING SHEARS TO CUT TWO MATCHING CIRCLES OF FABRIC THAT ARE 14 INCHES IN DIAMETER.

14"

2. STUFF THE TOES OF OLD STOCKINGS WITH FABRIC SCRAPS AND TIE WITH THREAD.

THREAD

3. COVER THE STUFFED STOCKINGS WITH CIRCLES OF CLOTH. GATHER THE EDGES TOGETHER AND TIE WITH RIBBON OR YARN.

4. INSERT DECORATIVE ORNAMENTS UNDER THE RIBBON.

Chapter Eight

CRAFT PROJECTS FOR USE BY AGENCIES

OUTREACH PROGRAMS

Level of difficulty: ****_-****

MATERIALS: A program, brochures or handouts about your organization, favors, props, sound system, and refreshments.

APPLICATIONS: Agencies and organizations are always looking for meaningful and entertaining programs.

PREPARATION BEFORE CRAFT SESSION: The main branch of your public library will have a listing of community organizations. Call the contact for selected organizations to see if there is any interest in reciprocal programming. Patients and staff may have contacts in the community who would be interested in a program. You may want to select a program from this book such as Music Day. The program can be enhanced by making your own props and musical instruments. Arrange transportation and refreshments.

CRAFT SESSION: Prepare projects for backdrops (see Murals), invitations (see Holiday Cards), and favors (see Wooden Horses). Design and rehearse a program (see Music Day). Have fun!

OUTREACH PROGRAMS

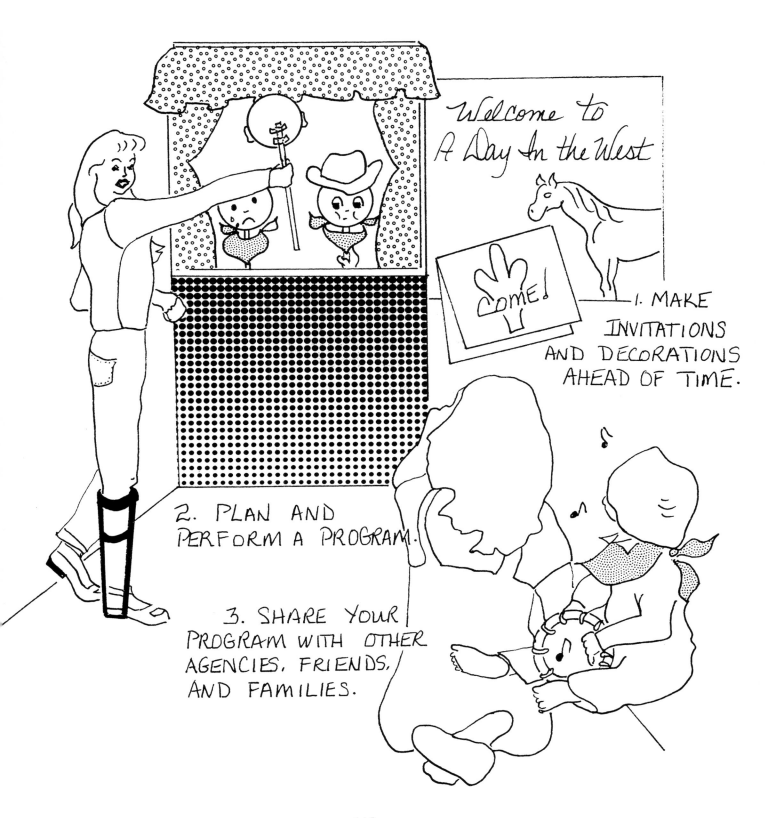

Welcome to
A Day In the West

Come!

1. MAKE INVITATIONS AND DECORATIONS AHEAD OF TIME.

2. PLAN AND PERFORM A PROGRAM.

3. SHARE YOUR PROGRAM WITH OTHER AGENCIES, FRIENDS, AND FAMILIES.

CALENDARS

Level of difficulty: *-*****

MATERIALS: 9 × 12 white or colored paper, drawing painting supplies, frames or mounting supplies, box and ballots, pencils.

APPLICATIONS: These calendars are a wonderful fund raiser for virtually any organization. An added benefit is media attention and publicity for your agency.

PREPARATION BEFORE CRAFT SESSION: Choose a theme for your calendar—seasonal, family, pets, etc. Printers or local businesses may be willing to financially underwrite publication of your calendar. It may be distributed through local banks, groceries, and bookstores. So many of the pictures will be lovely that your main problem may be in deciding which ones to include in the calendar. For added PR, frame and display all the art work in a local exhibition room (bank lobby, botanic gardens, library, etc.) and have a public ballot— complete with opening night reception and refreshments.

CRAFT SESSION: Have each participant create one or more paintings or drawings. Ask the participant for a title and brief descriptive statement. Note the title and artist's name on each piece. You may want to include the descriptive statements on cards at the exhibition.

CALENDARS

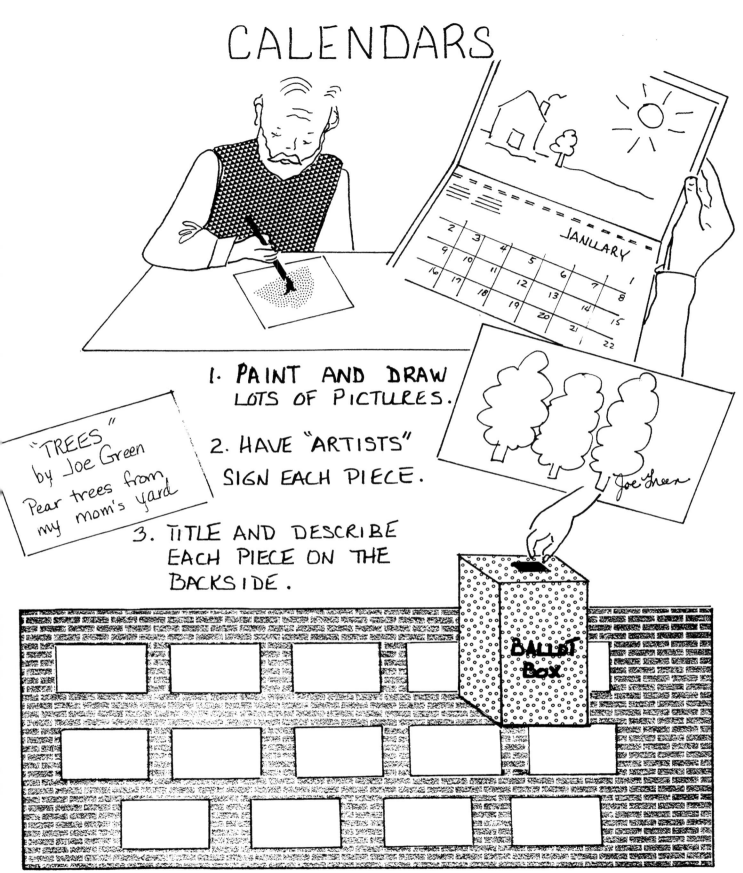

1. PAINT AND DRAW LOTS OF PICTURES.

2. HAVE "ARTISTS" SIGN EACH PIECE.

3. TITLE AND DESCRIBE EACH PIECE ON THE BACKSIDE.

"TREES"
by Joe Green
Pear trees from my mom's yard

JANUARY

BALLOT BOX

Joe Green

4. HAVE A PUBLIC BALLOT TO SELECT 12 PICTURES FOR YOUR CALENDAR.

TOY ANIMALS AND TOY BUILDINGS

Level of difficulty: ***-*****

MATERIALS: Wood scraps, 00 sandpaper, craft glue, water base paint in a variety of colors, brushes, felt marking pens.

APPLICATIONS: These imaginative toys are appreciated during the holiday season by volunteer agencies and by community clubs that sponsor programs for the needy. You can also donate the toys to the Salvation Army or to church nurseries. This is a great project for men, women, and children alike.

PREPARATION BEFORE CRAFT SESSION: You may want to glue together some animals or buildings for those people who do not want to wait for glue to dry before painting. See craft session for instructions.

CRAFT SESSION: Pick out some interesting pieces of wood that look somewhat like animal shapes or parts of buildings. Fit the pieces together to create imaginary animals or buildings. After you have selected the pieces of wood, sand them all smooth with 00 sandpaper. Then fit the parts together again, and glue them in place. Paint them any colors you wish. Allow this first coat of paint to dry. Then use paint or felt pens to draw detail designs with other colors. Do this very free hand. Make lots of toys.

TOY ANIMALS

WOOD SCRAPS FROM
LUMBER YARD.

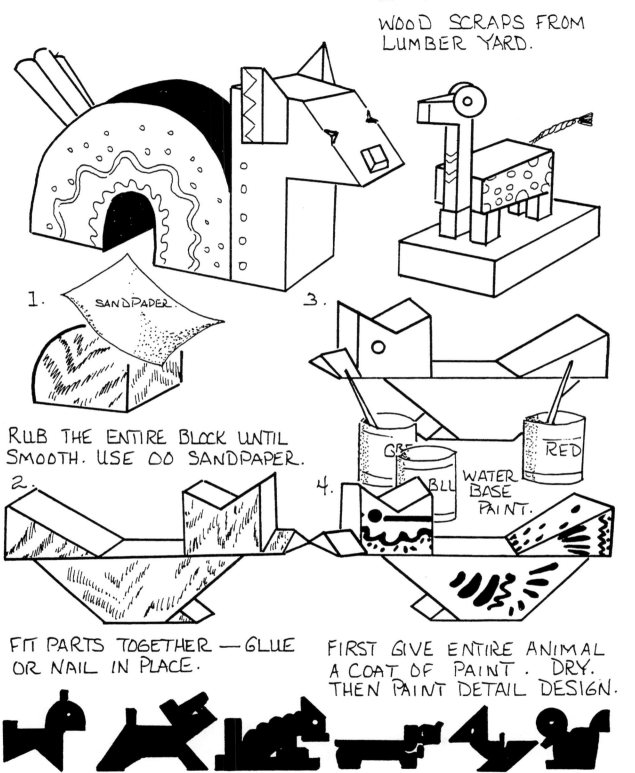

1. SANDPAPER

RUB THE ENTIRE BLOCK UNTIL
SMOOTH. USE OO SANDPAPER.

2. FIT PARTS TOGETHER — GLUE
OR NAIL IN PLACE.

3.

4. GREEN BLUE RED WATER
BASE
PAINT.

FIRST GIVE ENTIRE ANIMAL
A COAT OF PAINT. DRY.
THEN PAINT DETAIL DESIGN.

149

TOY BUILDINGS

USE WOOD SCRAPS
FOR THESE CREATIVE
TOYS AND MODELS.

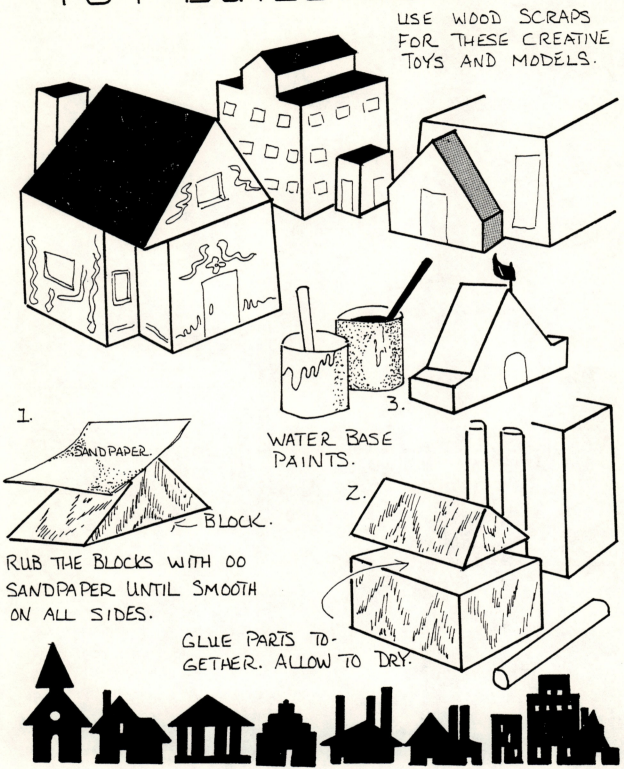

WATER BASE
PAINTS.

1. SANDPAPER. BLOCK.

RUB THE BLOCKS WITH OO
SANDPAPER UNTIL SMOOTH
ON ALL SIDES.

2.

3.

GLUE PARTS TO-
GETHER. ALLOW TO DRY.

TREE TRIMMING

Level of difficulty: *-*****

MATERIALS: Colored or white art paper of a medium or heavy weight, scissors, string, narrow ribbon, craft glue, brushes, crayons, felt marking pens in a variety of colors, glue stick, paper punch (metallic paper, gold and silver stars, lace—all optional).

APPLICATIONS: These holiday ornaments may be donated by the dozens to nursing homes or to your local volunteer bureau.

PREPARATION BEFORE CRAFT SESSION: Cut out dozens of patterns. Distribute one of each design in front of each person and secure them to the table with glue stick.

CRAFT SESSION: Decorate the patterns with crayon or felt markers. Sign each pattern when complete. Follow the directions on the charts for folding and gluing. Add gold and silver stars, lace, and ribbons if you wish, or make the stars of metallic paper, or metallic wallpaper scraps.

TREE TRIMMING BIRDS

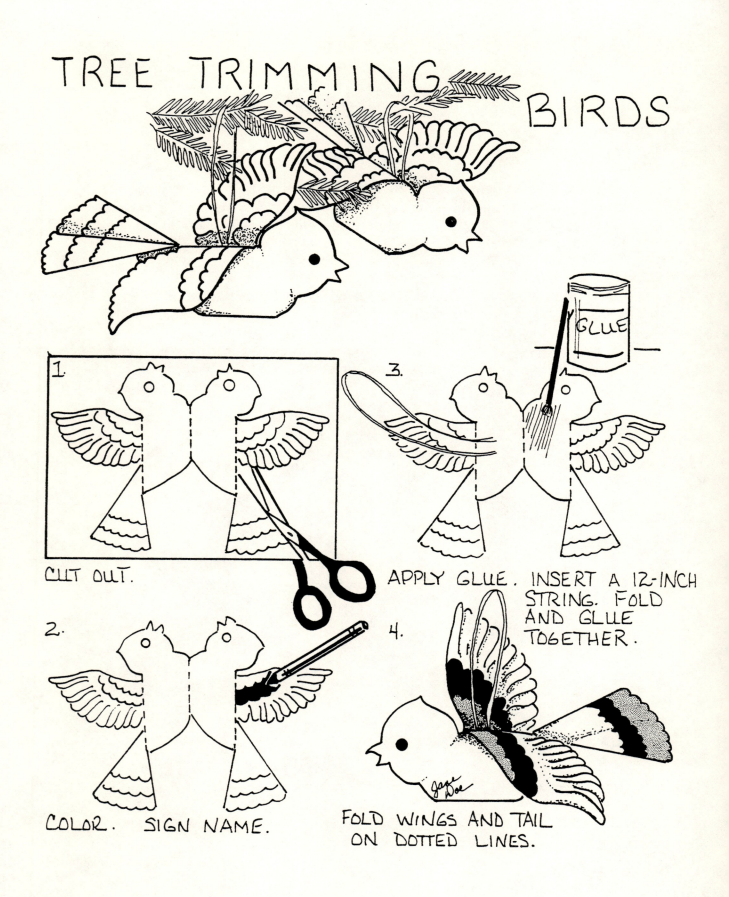

1. CUT OUT.

2. COLOR. SIGN NAME.

3. APPLY GLUE. INSERT A 12-INCH STRING. FOLD AND GLUE TOGETHER.

4. FOLD WINGS AND TAIL ON DOTTED LINES.

PATTERN FOR TREE TRIMMING.
BIRDS

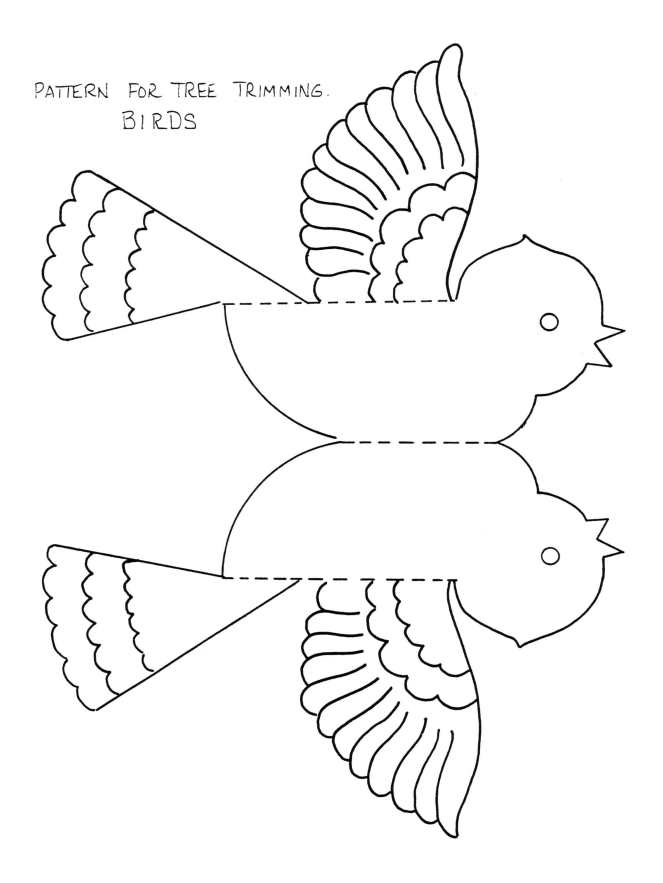

TREE ANGEL

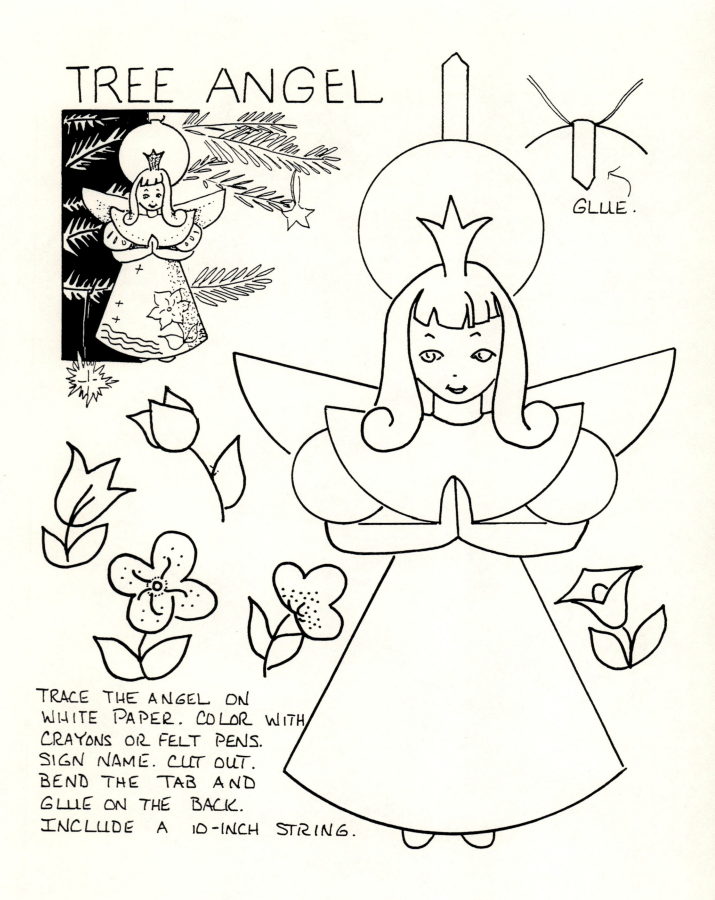

GLUE.

TRACE THE ANGEL ON
WHITE PAPER. COLOR WITH
CRAYONS OR FELT PENS.
SIGN NAME. CUT OUT.
BEND THE TAB AND
GLUE ON THE BACK.
INCLUDE A 10-INCH STRING.

TREE ANGEL

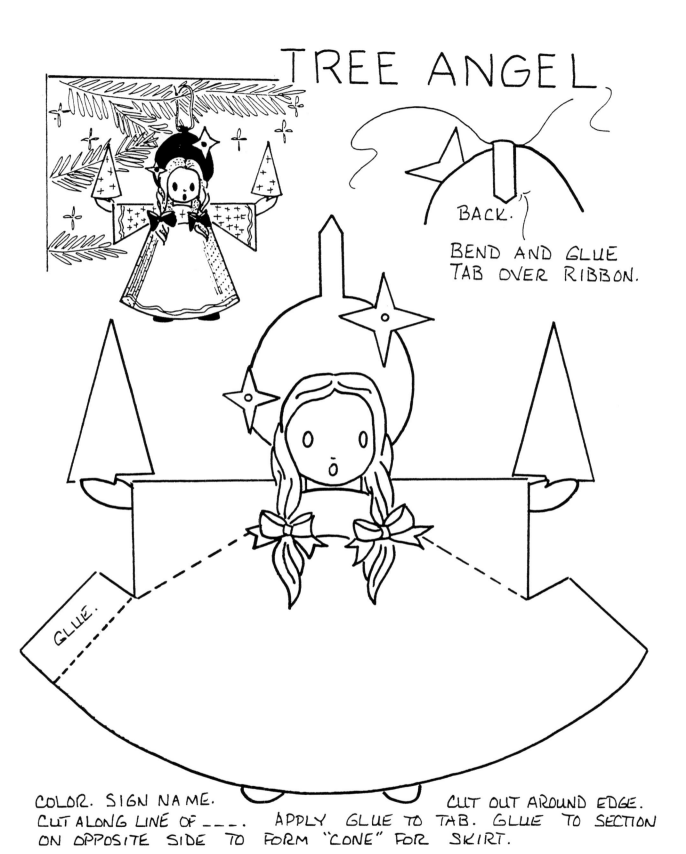

BACK.

BEND AND GLUE
TAB OVER RIBBON.

GLUE.

COLOR. SIGN NAME.   CUT OUT AROUND EDGE.
CUT ALONG LINE OF ___.   APPLY GLUE TO TAB. GLUE TO SECTION
ON OPPOSITE SIDE TO FORM "CONE" FOR SKIRT.

PAPER STARS

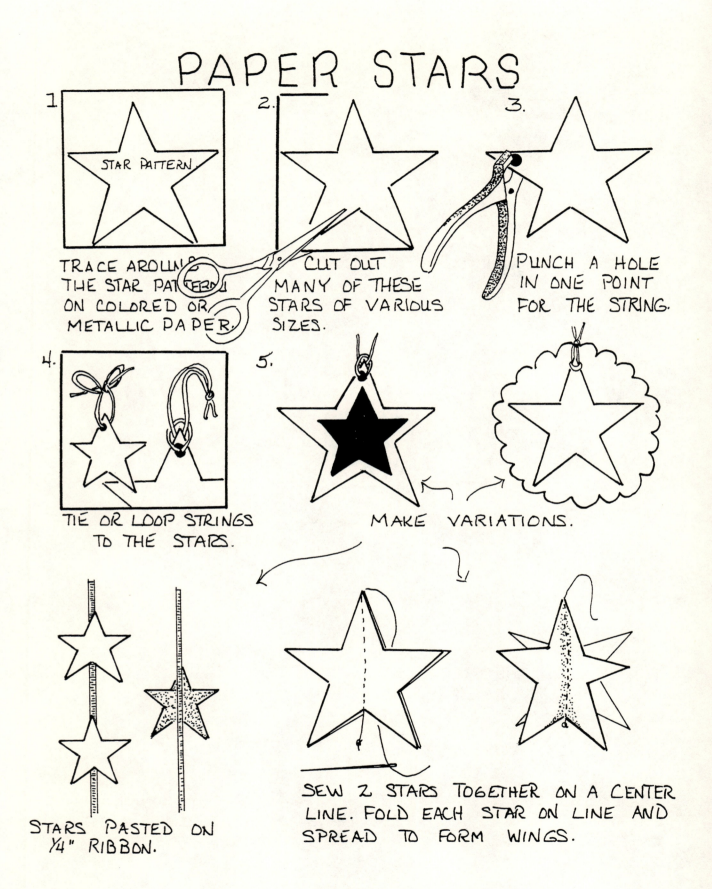

1. STAR PATTERN

TRACE AROUND THE STAR PATTERN ON COLORED OR METALLIC PAPER.

2. CUT OUT MANY OF THESE STARS OF VARIOUS SIZES.

3. PUNCH A HOLE IN ONE POINT FOR THE STRING.

4. TIE OR LOOP STRINGS TO THE STARS.

5. MAKE VARIATIONS.

STARS PASTED ON ¼" RIBBON.

SEW 2 STARS TOGETHER ON A CENTER LINE. FOLD EACH STAR ON LINE AND SPREAD TO FORM WINGS.

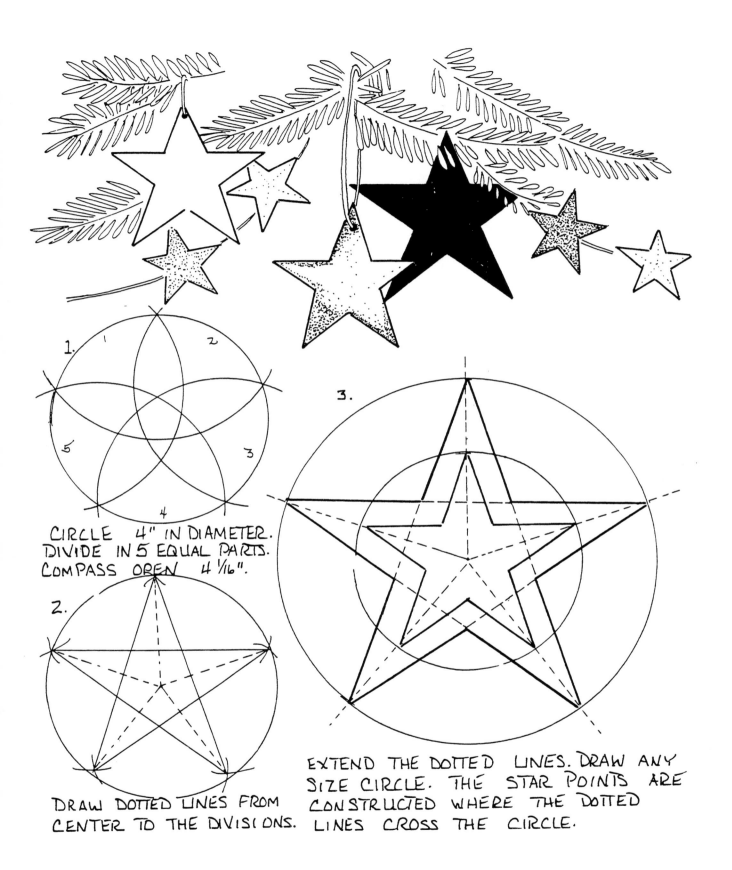

1.

CIRCLE 4" IN DIAMETER.
DIVIDE IN 5 EQUAL PARTS.
COMPASS OPEN 4 1/16".

2.

DRAW DOTTED LINES FROM
CENTER TO THE DIVISIONS.

3.

EXTEND THE DOTTED LINES. DRAW ANY
SIZE CIRCLE. THE STAR POINTS ARE
CONSTRUCTED WHERE THE DOTTED
LINES CROSS THE CIRCLE.

ORNAMENTS

Level of difficulty: *****

MATERIALS: Glitter, craft glue, empty margarine tubs, large sequins, straight pins, 6-inch Styrofoam ball, metallic ribbon or cord, empty medicine cups, scissors, wet paper towels or a wet washcloth or sponge.

APPLICATIONS: These ornaments are spectacular. Donate them to your local fire department and police station at holiday time to express appreciation for the expertise they demonstrate all year in help for the disabled and handicapped.

PREPARATION BEFORE CRAFT SESSION: Cut a piece of ribbon 24 inches long. Fold the ribbon in half to make a long loop, and secure it to the Styrofoam ball with glue. Sprinkle glitter over the excess glue for decoration. Pour glue into one margarine tub and glitter into another. Stick straight pins through the large sequins and put them in a margarine tub to hold for safekeeping.

CRAFT SESSION: Dip the rim of a medicine cup lightly in glue. Then dip it in glitter. Now dip the bottom of the same cup in glue and secure it on the Styrofoam ball with a straight pin and sequin. (Use thimble or eraser end on a pencil if your finger hurts.) Repeat this process until the entire ball is covered with medicine cups, which have been placed as close to each other as possible. Use the wet towels, sponge, or wash cloth whenever fingers get sticky.

ORNAMENTS

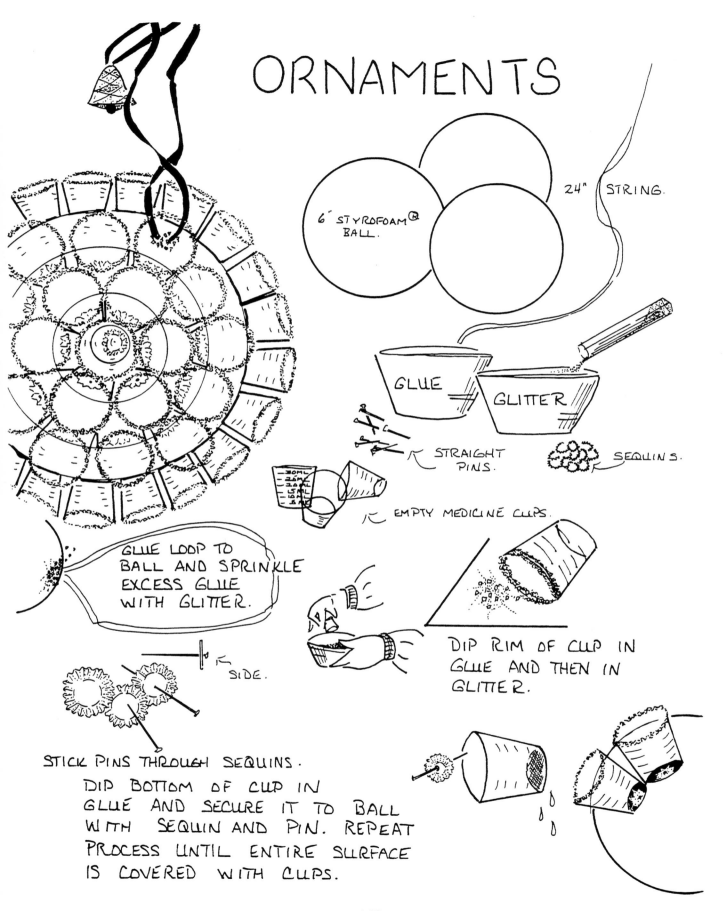

6" STYROFOAM® BALL.

24" STRING.

GLUE

GLITTER

STRAIGHT PINS.

SEQUINS.

EMPTY MEDICINE CUPS.

GLUE LOOP TO BALL AND SPRINKLE EXCESS GLUE WITH GLITTER.

DIP RIM OF CUP IN GLUE AND THEN IN GLITTER.

SIDE.

STICK PINS THROUGH SEQUINS.

DIP BOTTOM OF CUP IN GLUE AND SECURE IT TO BALL WITH SEQUIN AND PIN. REPEAT PROCESS UNTIL ENTIRE SURFACE IS COVERED WITH CUPS.

159

HOLIDAY CARDS

Level of difficulty: *-**

MATERIALS: Colored construction paper, felt marking pens, ribbon, glue stick, paper punch, scissors (holiday stickers, optional).

APPLICATIONS: These simple cards are appreciated by your governmental volunteer agency, which will distribute the cards on meal trays to hospitals and nursing homes.

PREPARATION BEFORE CRAFT SESSION: Cut ribbon into 12-inch lengths. Trace the outline of the pattern of the cards on a folded piece of construction paper. Cut it out double, but do not cut along the folded edge. Make an eyelet hole in the position indicated. Using glue stick, secure a card in front of each person.

CRAFT SESSION: Decorate the cards with felt pens. Some people may prefer to put holiday stickers on the cards rather than draw. Write greetings inside each card, and have the patients sign their names. Tie the cards with a 12-inch length of narrow ribbon.

HOLIDAY CARDS

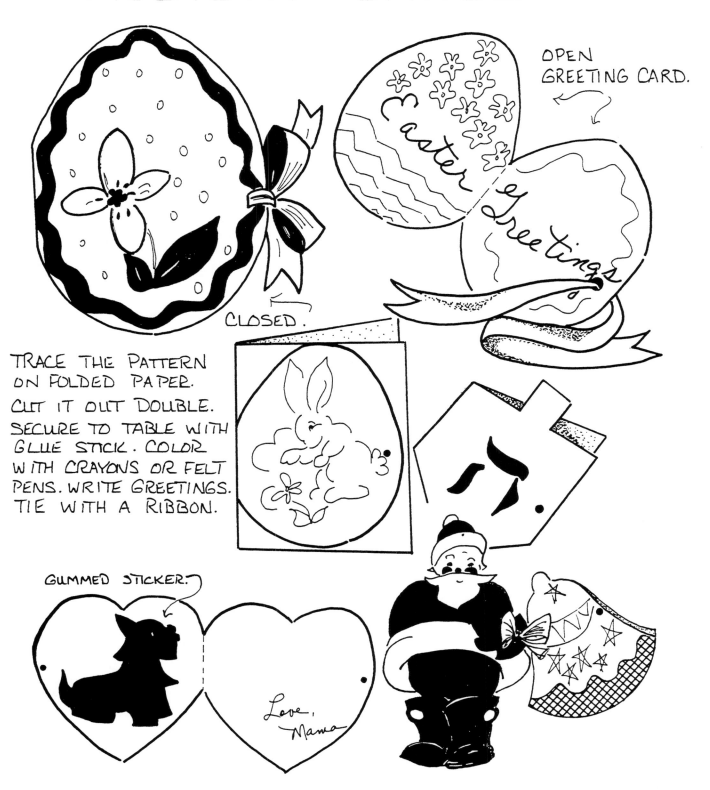

OPEN GREETING CARD.

Easter greetings

CLOSED.

TRACE THE PATTERN ON FOLDED PAPER. CUT IT OUT DOUBLE. SECURE TO TABLE WITH GLUE STICK. COLOR WITH CRAYONS OR FELT PENS. WRITE GREETINGS. TIE WITH A RIBBON.

GUMMED STICKER.

Love, Mama

EASTER

CENTER FOLD.

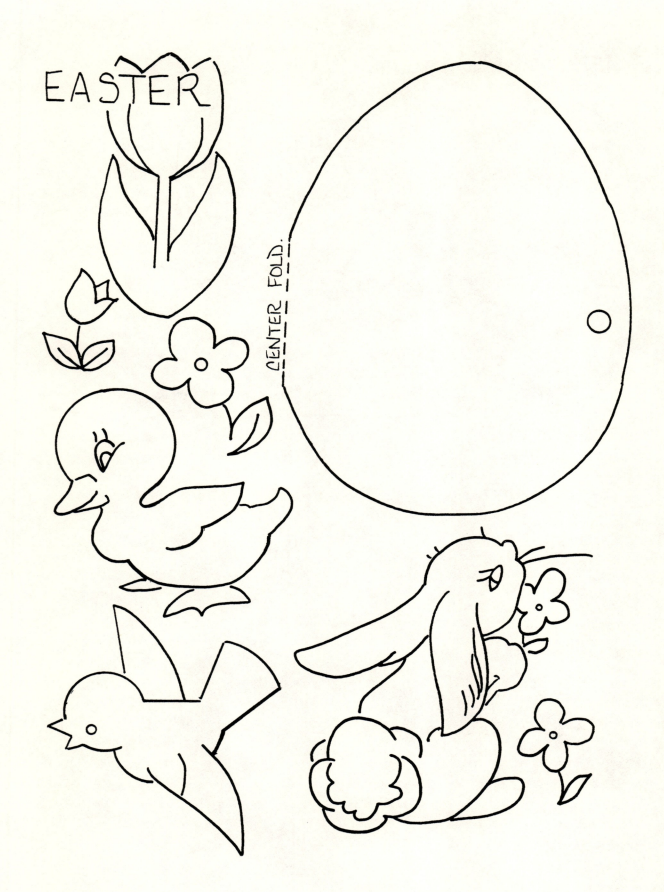

162

PASSOVER

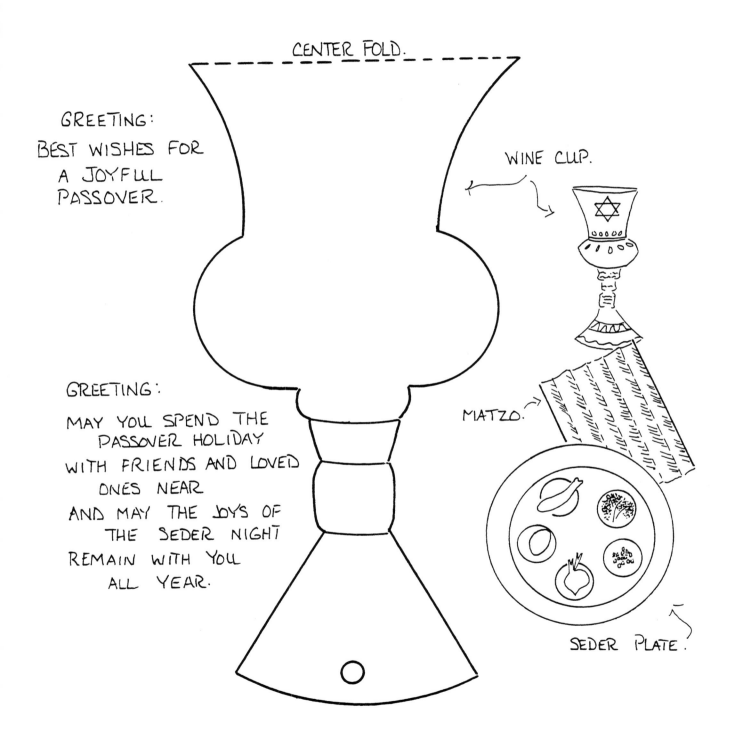

CENTER FOLD.

GREETING:
BEST WISHES FOR
A JOYFUL
PASSOVER.

WINE CUP.

GREETING:

MAY YOU SPEND THE
PASSOVER HOLIDAY
WITH FRIENDS AND LOVED
ONES NEAR
AND MAY THE JOYS OF
THE SEDER NIGHT
REMAIN WITH YOU
ALL YEAR.

MATZO.

SEDER PLATE.

VALENTINES DAY

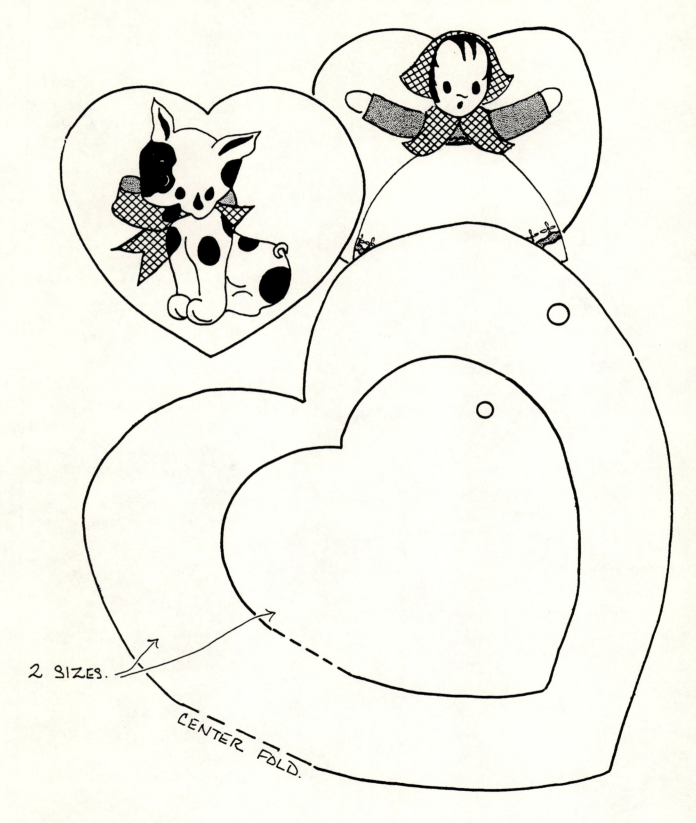

2 SIZES.

CENTER FOLD.

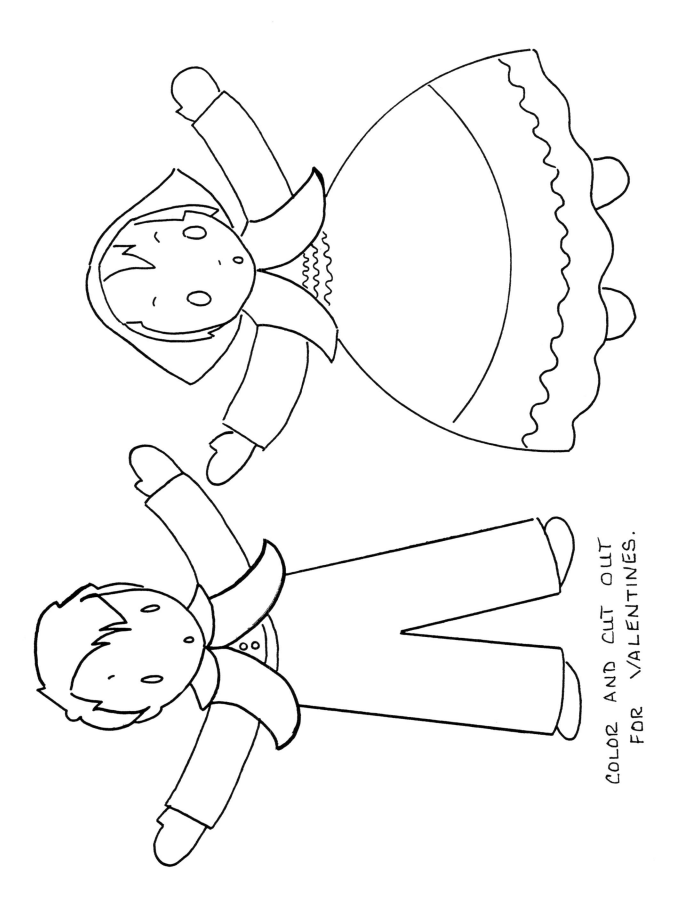

COLOR AND CUT OUT FOR VALENTINES.

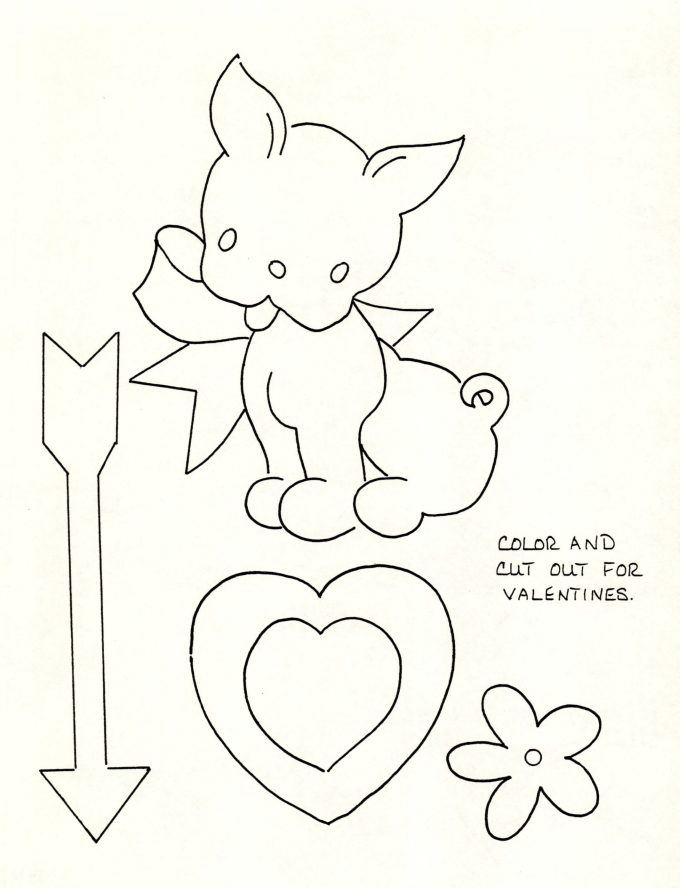

COLOR AND
CUT OUT FOR
VALENTINES.

CHRISTMAS

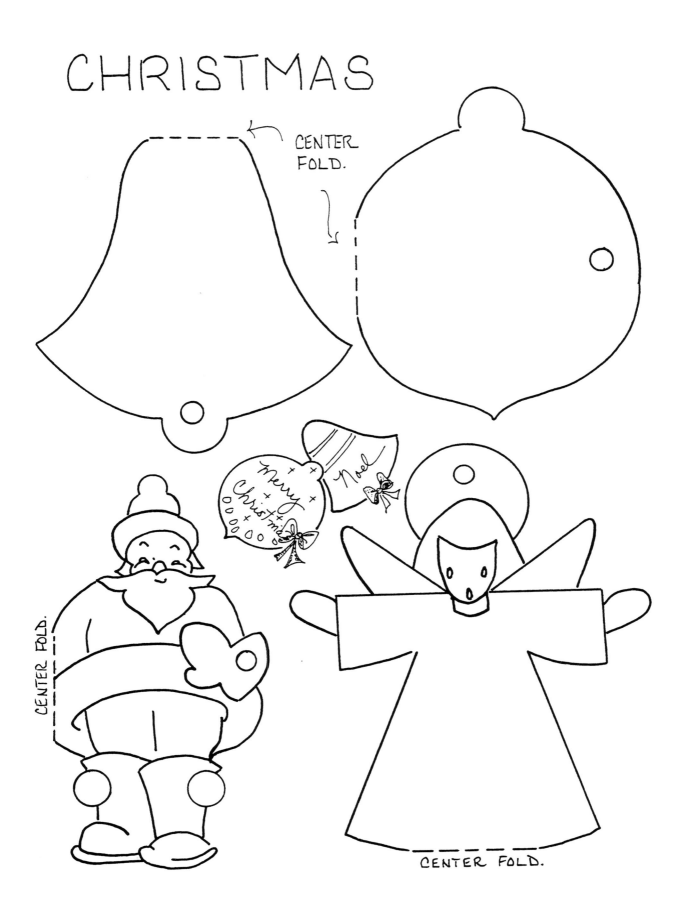

CENTER FOLD.

CENTER FOLD.

CENTER FOLD.

CHRISTMAS

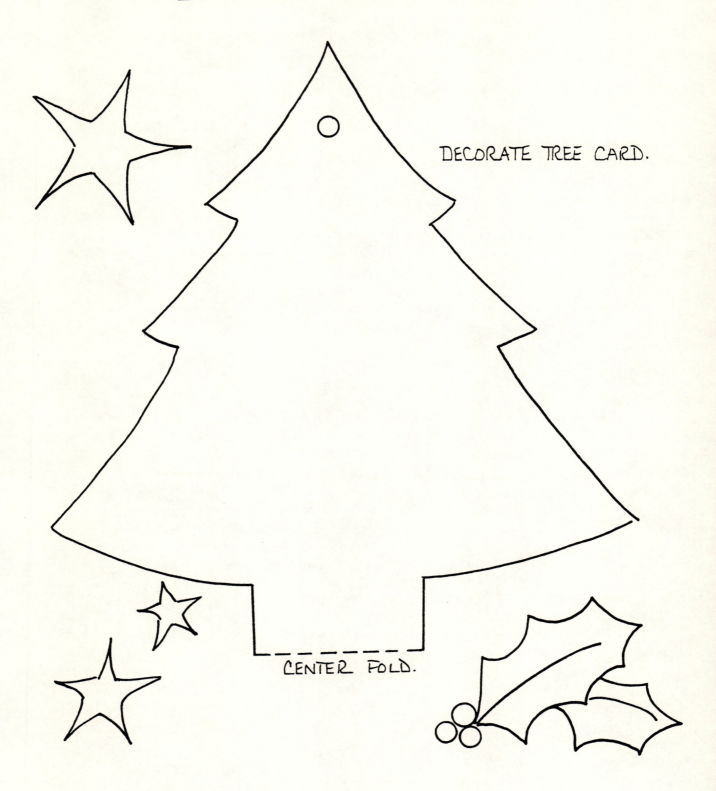

DECORATE TREE CARD.

CENTER FOLD.

CHANUKAH

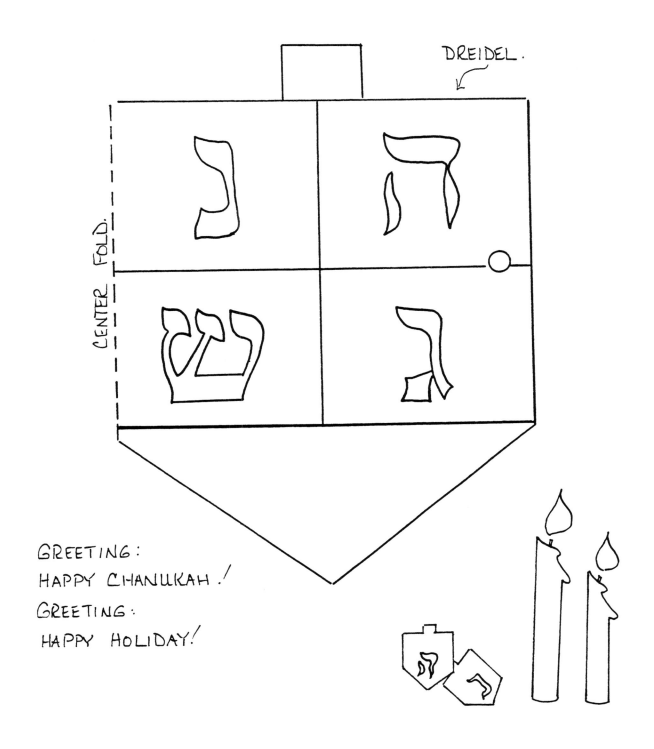

DREIDEL.

CENTER FOLD.

GREETING:
HAPPY CHANUKAH!
GREETING:
HAPPY HOLIDAY!

JEWISH NEW YEAR

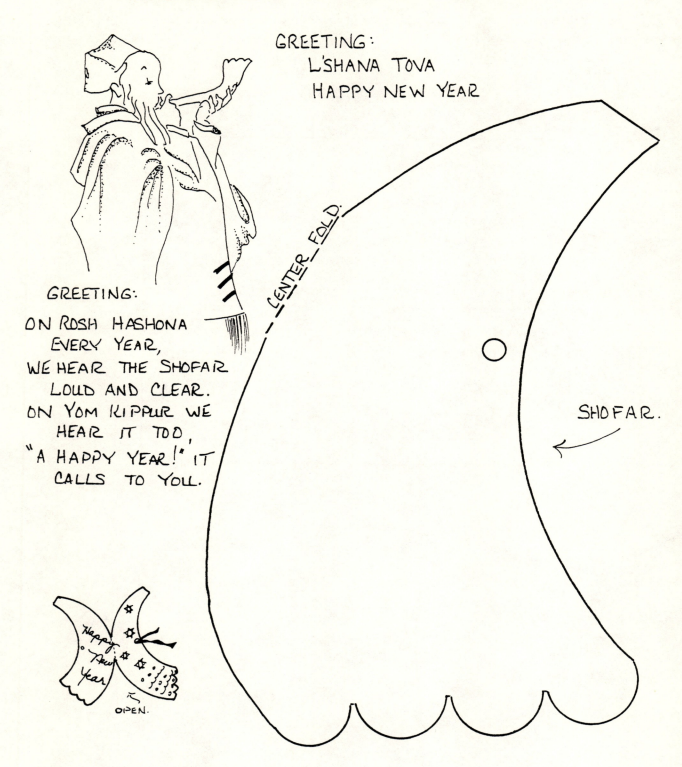

GREETING:
L'SHANA TOVA
HAPPY NEW YEAR

GREETING:

ON ROSH HASHONA
EVERY YEAR,
WE HEAR THE SHOFAR
LOUD AND CLEAR.
ON YOM KIPPUR WE
HEAR IT TOO,
"A HAPPY YEAR!" IT
CALLS TO YOU.

CENTER FOLD.

SHOFAR.

Happy New Year

OPEN.

SCISSORS CAN

Level of difficulty: *-***

MATERIALS: Fabric scraps, pinking shears, craft glue, brushes, empty 16 ounce frozen concentrated juice cans (makes 1/2 gallon), ric rac or ball fringe.

APPLICATIONS: Any government agency can use lots of scissors cans for secretaries' desks. The nice tall height of this size juice can makes a very stable container which holds lots of scissors and will not tip over. (We carry these around in our supply box so we do not have to dig to find our shears.) You might want to donate pretty cans to fabric stores which would in turn supply you with samples or remnants. Note that these cans are useful for pencils, combs, paintbrushes, straws, etc.

PREPARATION BEFORE CRAFT SESSION: Using a pinking shears, cut fabric into pieces 61/4 inches by 9 inches.

CRAFT SESSION: Brush glue on the can. Wrap fabric around the can. Decorate the top with ric rac or fringe.

SCISSORS CAN

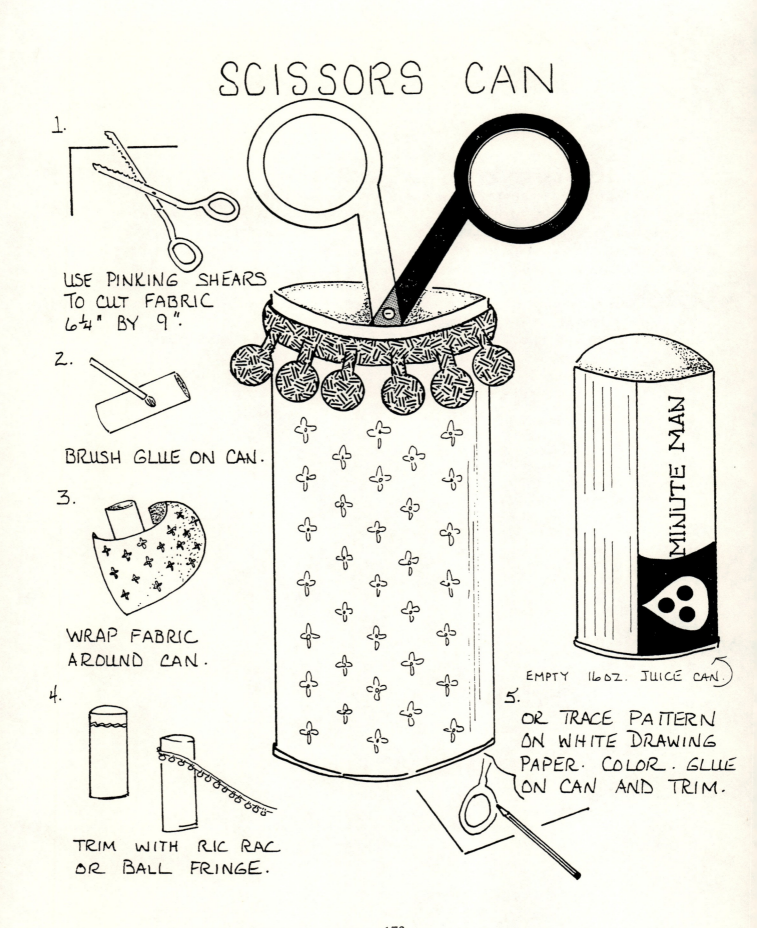

1. USE PINKING SHEARS TO CUT FABRIC 6¼" BY 9".

2. BRUSH GLUE ON CAN.

3. WRAP FABRIC AROUND CAN.

4. TRIM WITH RIC RAC OR BALL FRINGE.

MINUTE MAN

EMPTY 16 OZ. JUICE CAN.

5. OR TRACE PATTERN ON WHITE DRAWING PAPER. COLOR. GLUE ON CAN AND TRIM.

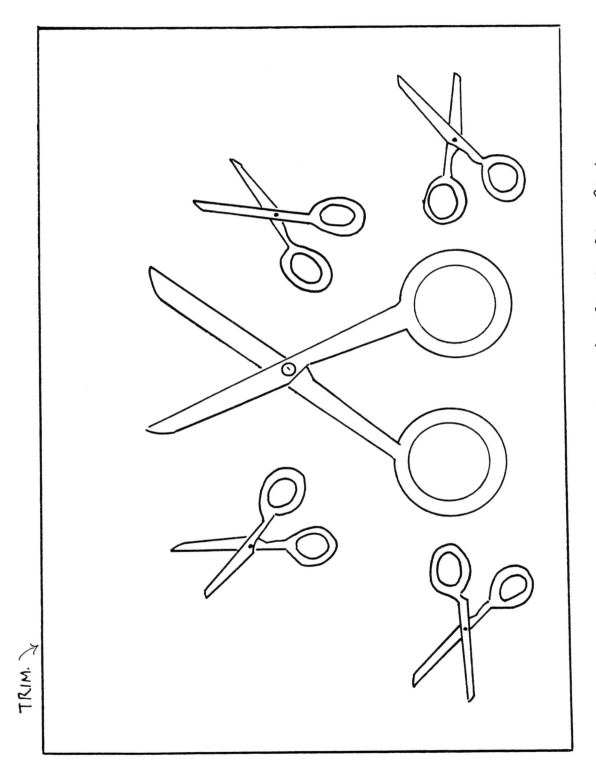

TRIM.

PATTERN FOR PAPER-COVERED SCISSORS CAN.

173

JINGLES AND JANGLES

Level of difficulty: ***-*****

MATERIALS: Package handles, fine wire, hammer, small pieces of plywood (optional), bottle caps, nails, rattles, bells, or soft drink pull tabs.

APPLICATIONS: These musical jingles and jangles are enjoyable both to make and use. They are grand for nursing home rhythm bands, family service agencies or orphanages, and government daycare and preschool programs. Men especially will like to do the hammer and nail work in making these.

PREPARATION BEFORE CRAFT SESSION: For each package handle, flatten six or eight bottle caps by tapping the edges down toward the outside with a hammer. Cut the wire into six-inch lengths. Leave some bottle caps unprepared for those people who are able to flatten them.

CRAFT SESSION: If you are not working on a work table or bench, place the caps on plywood. Then with a hammer and nail, punch a hole in the center of each bottle cap. Fasten the end of the wire to one side of the package handle, string the bottle caps on the wire, and fasten the end of the wire to the opposite side of the package handle. Shake the handles for jingles and jangles. Try various metallic objects like nails, bells, screws, pull tabs, and rattles instead of bottle caps.

JINGLES AND JANGLES

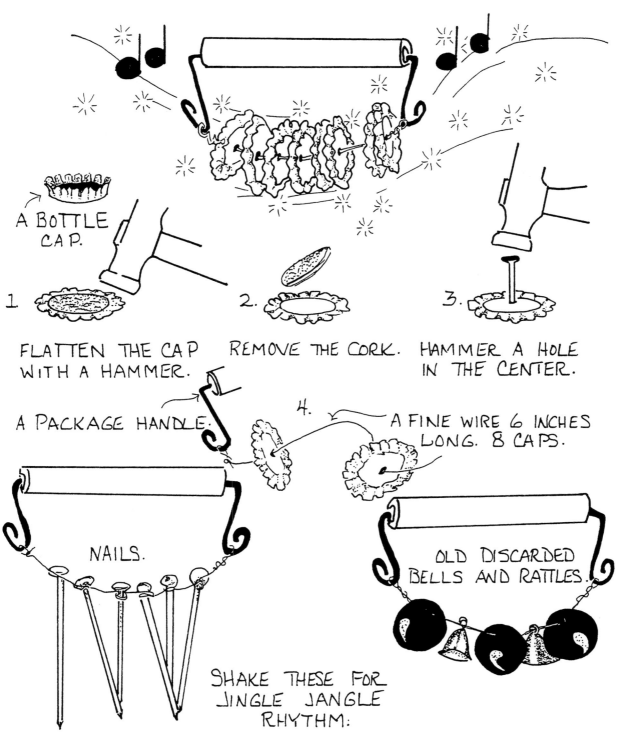

A BOTTLE CAP.

1. FLATTEN THE CAP WITH A HAMMER.

2. REMOVE THE CORK.

3. HAMMER A HOLE IN THE CENTER.

A PACKAGE HANDLE.

4. A FINE WIRE 6 INCHES LONG. 8 CAPS.

NAILS.

OLD DISCARDED BELLS AND RATTLES.

SHAKE THESE FOR JINGLE JANGLE RHYTHM:

BOOKMARKS

Level of difficulty: ***-*****

MATERIALS: Colored art paper, clear contact paper, scissors, pinking shears, paper punch, narrow satin ribbon (or bias binding, ric rac, etc.), dried flowers and leaves, straight pin, black felt marking pen, wax stick pick-up (available in jewelry section of craft stores.)

APPLICATIONS: The illustration shows how to make bookmarks by using materials from nature. After trying these, you can make interesting notepaper, pictures, etc. Donate the bookmarks to the public library or a nearby school.

PREPARATION BEFORE CRAFT SESSION: Cut 2 × 6 inch strips of colored art paper. For each strip of paper, cut two pieces of contact paper the same size. Also cut 12-inch strips of narrow ribbon. Have a nice collection of dried blossoms, leaves, weeds, or ferns. To dry plants, place the picked leaves or blossoms (preferably flat ones) in an old phone book or paperback or between sheets of newspaper. Let them stay untouched for one week. They will then be ready for use. Generally, have twice as much as is needed, because the delicate dried leaves and blossoms are easily broken. A wax stick may be used to make assembly easier. Clover and ferns are especially nice.

CRAFT SESSION: Have each person choose the color of paper he desires and the dried flowers and leaves he likes. Then have the individual arrange the flowers in a pleasing design and sign his name. Help him peel the contact paper and press it down on the leaves and paper. Use a pin to puncture the contact paper to get out any air bubbles. Repeat the design process on the other side. Trim all four edges with a pinking shears. Punch a hole at one end with a paper punch. Insert a ribbon by folding it in half and looping it through the hole.

BOOKMARKS

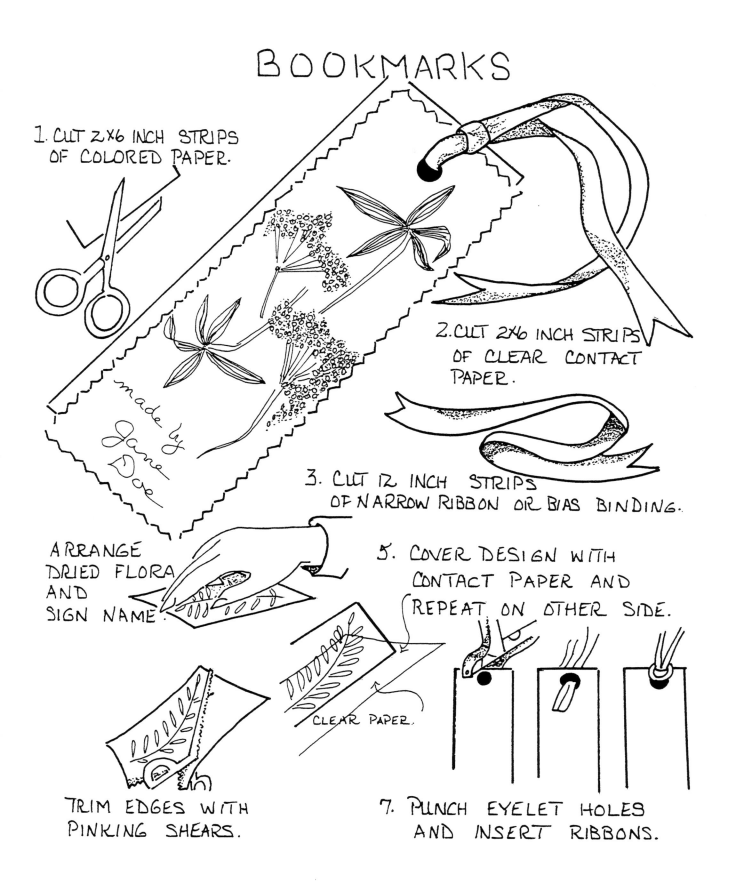

1. CUT 2X6 INCH STRIPS OF COLORED PAPER.

made by Jane Doe

2. CUT 2X6 INCH STRIPS OF CLEAR CONTACT PAPER.

3. CUT 12 INCH STRIPS OF NARROW RIBBON OR BIAS BINDING.

ARRANGE DRIED FLORA AND SIGN NAME.

5. COVER DESIGN WITH CONTACT PAPER AND REPEAT ON OTHER SIDE.

CLEAR PAPER.

TRIM EDGES WITH PINKING SHEARS.

7. PUNCH EYELET HOLES AND INSERT RIBBONS.

NUT BASKETS

Level of difficulty: ***-*****

MATERIALS: Colored construction paper, white drawing paper, crayons markers, or paint, scissors, glue, nuts, glue stick.

APPLICATIONS: Send these little Thanksgiving baskets to a local governmental volunteer agency for distribution to needy families.

PREPARATION BEFORE CRAFT SESSION: Cut the square pattern out of some heavy colored paper. Cut on the heavy line; mark the broken lines and shaded area. Cut out turkey or apples of white paper. Using glue stick, secure turkeys and apples to the table in front of each person.

CRAFT SESSION: Fold the squares to form a box. Do this by always folding towards the center and slipping the shaded squares toward the outside. Apply glue to the shaded areas and form the shape of a box. Color the apples and turkeys, and glue them to the sides of the box. Fill the baskets with nuts.

NUT BASKET

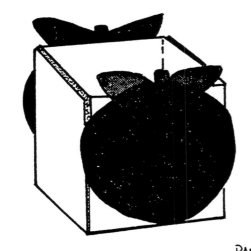

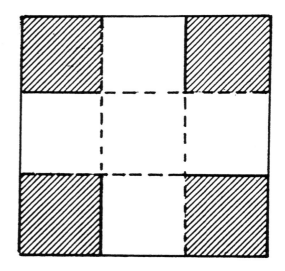

CUT THIS SQUARE PATTERN
OF HEAVY COLORED PAPER.
CUT ON HEAVY LINE ———.
FOLD ON BROKEN LINE ___.
APPLY GLUE ON SHADED
AREA ////.

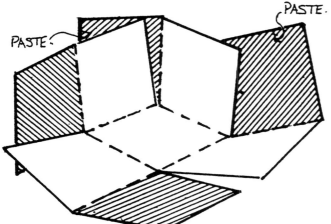

PASTE.

PASTE.

PASTE.

FOLD THE SQUARES TO FORM
A BOX. THE FOLDING IS ALWAYS
TOWARD THE CENTER. THE
GLUED SQUARES SLIP TO THE
OUTSIDE. THEN PRESS FIRMLY.

GLUE THE TURKEYS TO
THE BOX. FILL WITH
NUTS.

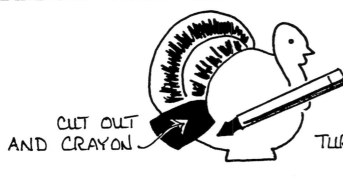

CUT OUT
AND CRAYON

TURKEYS OR APPLES.

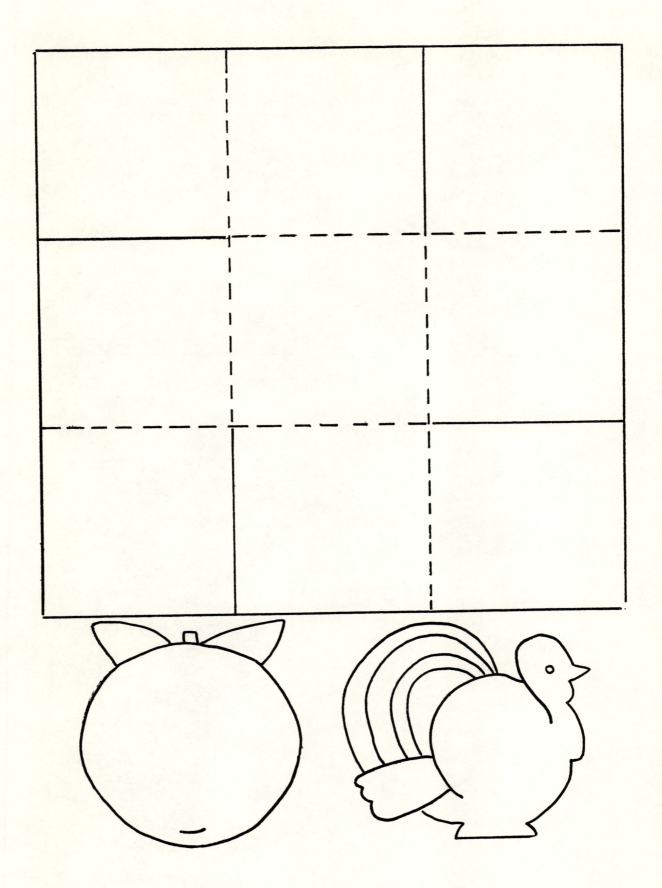

COASTERS

Level of difficulty: *-**

MATERIALS: Sample linoleum or formica tiles (at least 3 inches square), felt, craft glue, art paper, paper punch, crayons, black felt marking pen, glue stick, brush, magazine pictures (optional), water-based polyurethane (optional).

APPLICATIONS: These colorful coasters are nice for meal trays. You might send some sample coasters to your local radio stations for public service announcements to explain what some disabled people do for others who are also disabled.

PREPARATION BEFORE CRAFT SESSION: Cut art paper into 4½ inch squares. Trace patterns with black felt pens. Using glue stick, secure several squares in front of each person. Also, cut 4 felt corners for each tile.

CRAFT SESSION: Glue a piece of felt on each corner on the backs of the tiles. This gives the coasters a more finished look. Then have each person color his pattern with crayons. Remove the patterns from the table and help cut out the actual picture. Use a paper punch to cut eyes and flower centers. Then glue the pictures to the tiles. Some people prefer to cut out pictures from magazines to glue on the tiles. They are pretty, too. If you want the coasters to be waterproof, brush a layer of polyurethane on the completed tile.

COASTERS

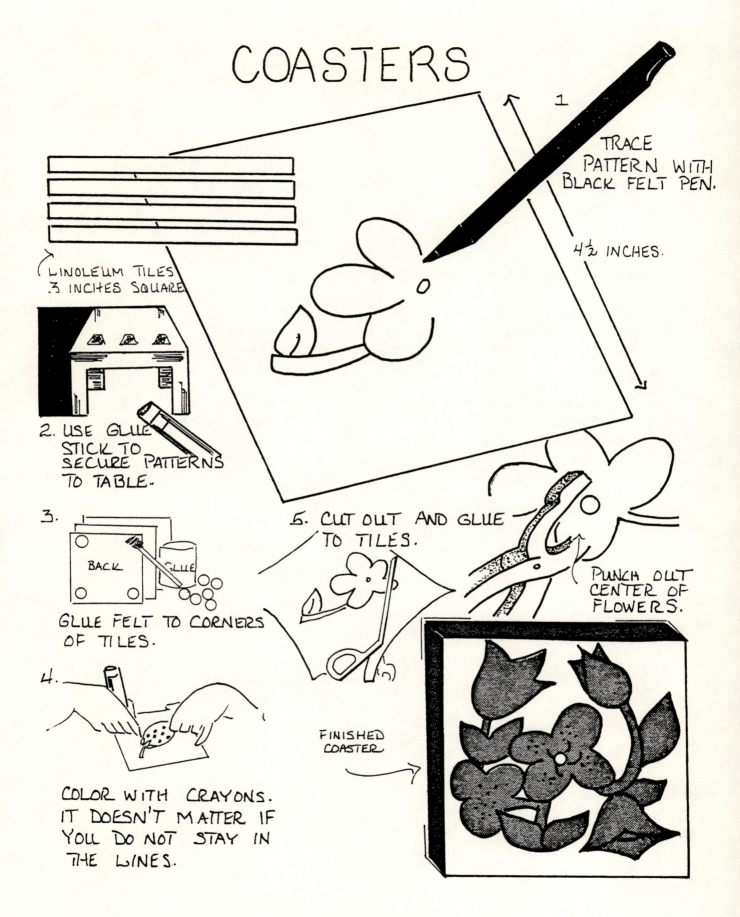

1. TRACE PATTERN WITH BLACK FELT PEN.

4½ INCHES.

LINOLEUM TILES 3 INCHES SQUARE.

2. USE GLUE STICK TO SECURE PATTERNS TO TABLE.

3. BACK GLUE

GLUE FELT TO CORNERS OF TILES.

4. COLOR WITH CRAYONS. IT DOESN'T MATTER IF YOU DO NOT STAY IN THE LINES.

5. CUT OUT AND GLUE TO TILES.

PUNCH OUT CENTER OF FLOWERS.

FINISHED COASTER

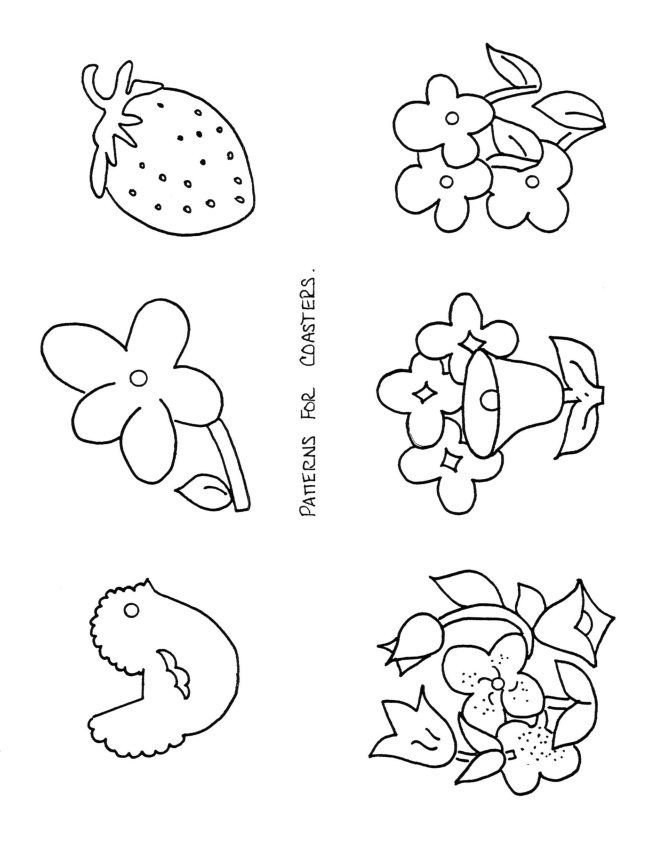

PATTERNS FOR COASTERS.

POTATO PRINT CARDS

Level of difficulty: *-*****

MATERIALS: Potatoes, knife, red and blue ink pads, white construction paper, ribbon or bias binding (red, white, and blue), felt marking pens (red and blue), paper punch, glue stick.

APPLICATIONS: These simple but eye-catching cards are particularly powerful when sent on the Fourth of July to city, state, and national government representatives to encourage legislation for the disabled and elderly. (Our nursing home had our congressman present a group of cards to the President welcoming him upon arrival to our city. We received a most grateful letter of appreciation.) The League of Women Voters will provide a list of names, titles, and addresses of all elected officials in government. Most officials personally answer mail, and this is especially exciting to residents of an institution or nursing home.

PREPARATION BEFORE CRAFT SESSION: Cut the potatoes in half. Draw a pattern on each half. Then cut the potato away from the pattern, leaving a relief (raised) design on the potato. Fold each piece of paper in half and punch three eyelet holes in each card along the unfolded edge. Cut the ribbon in 12-inch lengths. Using a glue stick, secure a card in front of each person.

CRAFT SESSION: Have each person press the potato on an ink pad and then on this paper. Be careful to keep colors separate. The more frequently the process is repeated, the more attractive is the card. Do not hesitate to overlap pressings of the potato stamp. Then finish decorating the cards with red and blue pens. Write greetings or messages or just sign signatures. Secure the cards with red, white, and blue ribbons looped through the three eyelets in each card.

POTATO PRINT CARDS

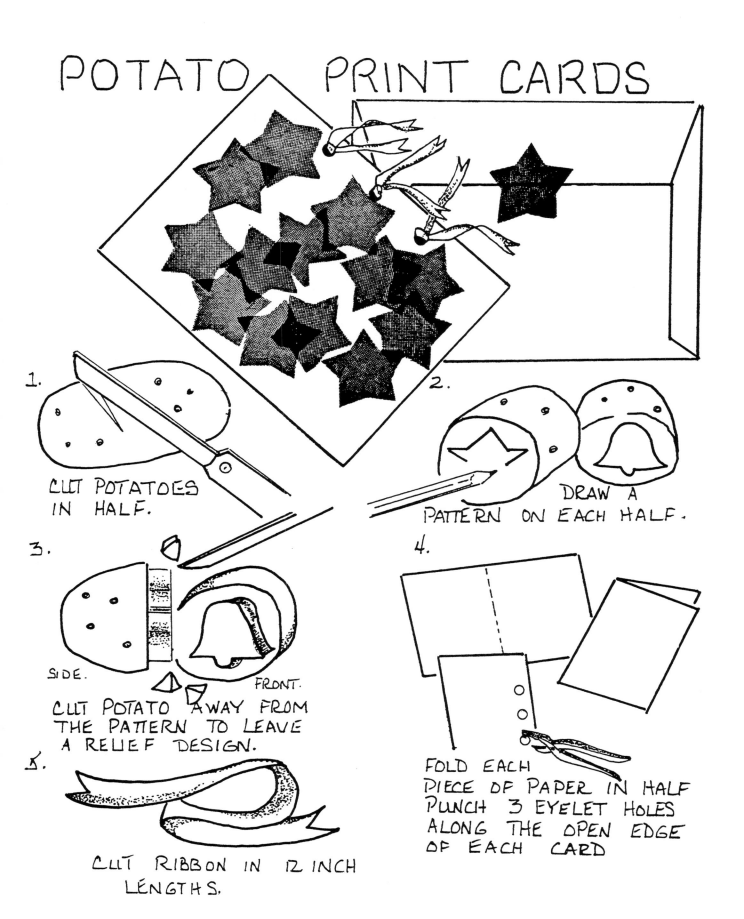

1. CUT POTATOES IN HALF.

2. DRAW A PATTERN ON EACH HALF.

3. SIDE. FRONT. CUT POTATO AWAY FROM THE PATTERN TO LEAVE A RELIEF DESIGN.

4. FOLD EACH PIECE OF PAPER IN HALF PUNCH 3 EYELET HOLES ALONG THE OPEN EDGE OF EACH CARD

5. CUT RIBBON IN 12 INCH LENGTHS.

POTATO PRINT CARDS

6.

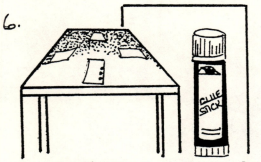

USE GLUE STICK TO SECURE A CARD IN FRONT OF EACH PERSON.

7.

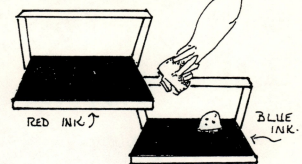

RED INK

BLUE INK.

PRESS POTATO DESIGN ON AN INK PAD.

8.

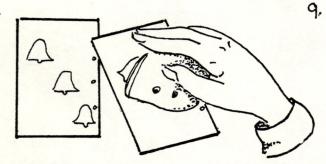

THEN PRESS THE INK COVERED POTATO ON THE PAPER. REPEAT PROCESS MANY TIMES.

PATTERNS FOR CARDS

9.

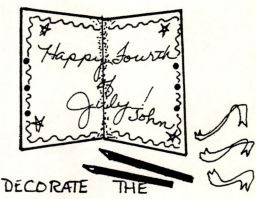

DECORATE THE INSIDE WITH RED AND BLUE FELT PENS. SIGN NAME AND TIE CLOSED. USE RED, WHITE, AND BLUE RIBBONS.

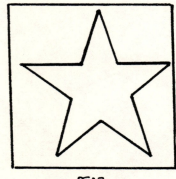

STAR.

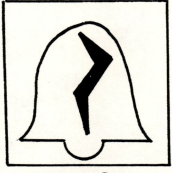

LIBERTY BELL.
(IF DESIRED, GOUGE OUT CRACK IN BELL.)

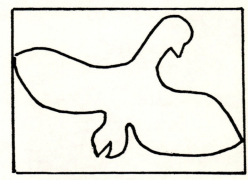

BALD EAGLE.

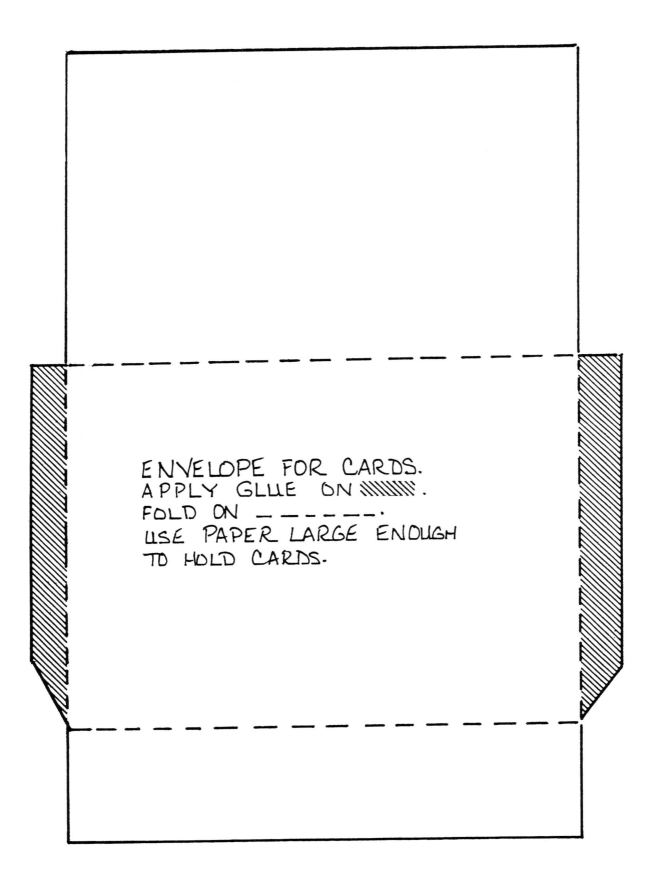

ENVELOPE FOR CARDS.
APPLY GLUE ON ░░░░░.
FOLD ON _ _ _ _ _ _ _ .
USE PAPER LARGE ENOUGH
TO HOLD CARDS.

Chapter Nine
CRAFT PROJECTS TO SELL

PAPER PLATE PUPPETS

Level of difficulty: *-*****

MATERIALS: White paper plates, cotton, glue, colored papers, feathers, pipe cleaners, felt, yarn, ribbon, glitter, sequins, 12″ to 18″ dowel sticks, masking tape, colored markers, scissors.

APPLICATIONS: Paper plate puppets can be sold as holiday decorations, toys, and they can be used for drama activities.

PREPARATION BEFORE CRAFT SESSION: Mark crosses for eyes, nose, and mouth on paper plates. Cut facial features out of colored paper and/or felt.

CRAFT SESSION: Decorate the plates. Tape dowel rods on the back of each plate. You may want to create your own puppet show and use it for Outreach Programs.

PAPER PLATE PUPPETS

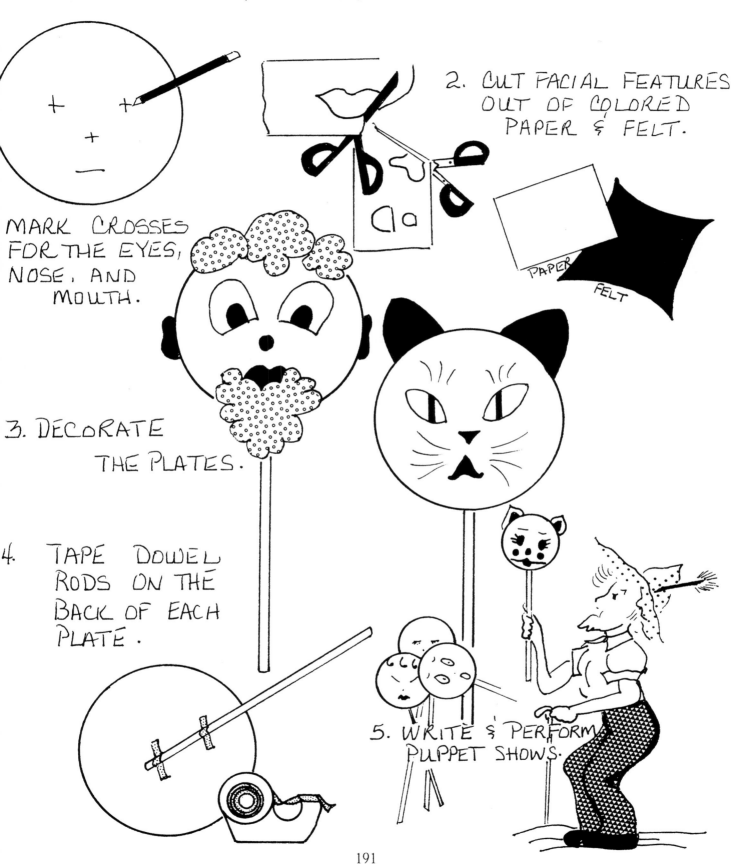

MARK CROSSES FOR THE EYES, NOSE, AND MOUTH.

2. CUT FACIAL FEATURES OUT OF COLORED PAPER & FELT.

PAPER

FELT

3. DECORATE THE PLATES.

4. TAPE DOWEL RODS ON THE BACK OF EACH PLATE.

5. WRITE & PERFORM PUPPET SHOWS.

TRIVETS

Level of difficulty: *-*****

MATERIALS: Lots of small mosaic tiles or bathroom tiles broken into small bits, craft glue, brush, grout, inexpensive metal hot pads or plastic lazy Susans, damp cloth, bowl and mixing utensil for the grout, water.

APPLICATIONS: These shiny hot pads are handy on any table. If you do not have a metal or plastic backing, just use a smooth board with felt glued on the back.

PREPARATION BEFORE CRAFT SESSION: None.

CRAFT SESSION: Place the tiles on a metal or plastic backing in any pattern or design you like. They should be spaced about 1/8 inch apart. Then glue them in place. When the glue is dry, mix the grout according to the package directions. Fill the cracks with grout and wipe the trivet clean with a damp cloth.

TRIVETS

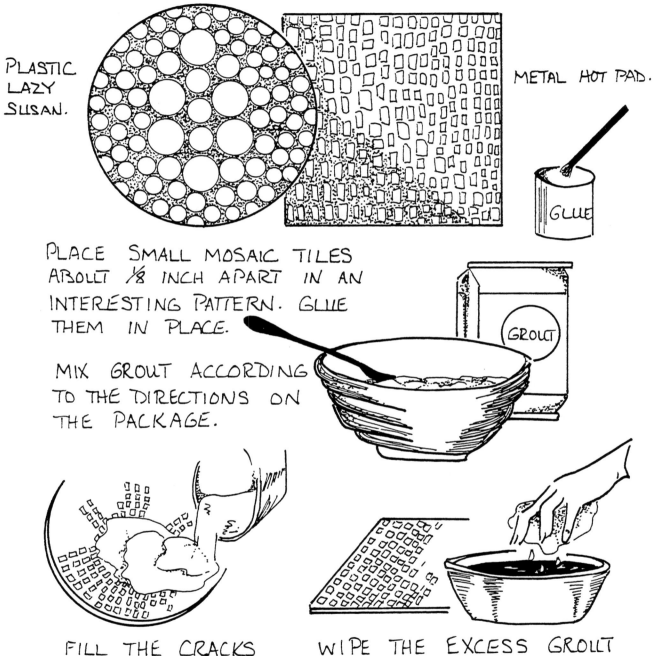

PLASTIC LAZY SUSAN.

METAL HOT PAD.

GLUE

PLACE SMALL MOSAIC TILES ABOUT ⅛ INCH APART IN AN INTERESTING PATTERN. GLUE THEM IN PLACE.

MIX GROUT ACCORDING TO THE DIRECTIONS ON THE PACKAGE.

GROUT

FILL THE CRACKS WITH GROUT.

WIPE THE EXCESS GROUT OFF THE TRIVET WITH A DAMP CLOTH.

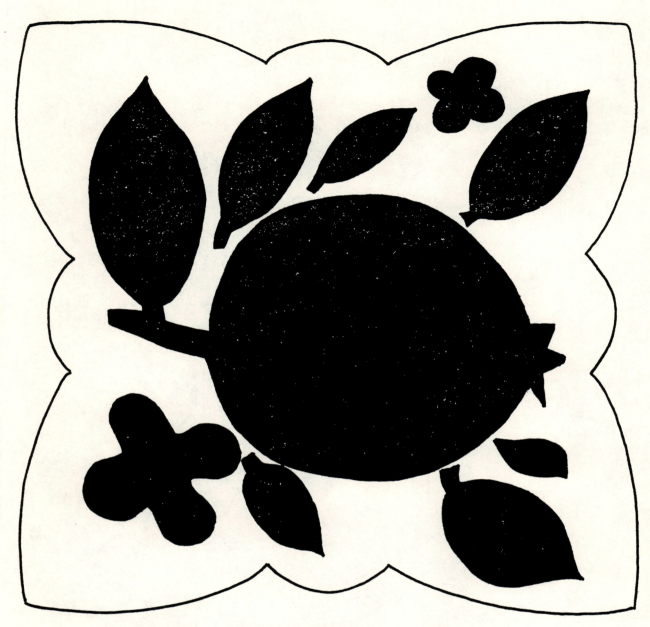

PATTERN FOR TRIVET MADE ON A
WOODEN BOARD. FILL IN THE BLACK
SILHOUETTE WITH TILE BITS OF ONE
COLOR, AND THE BACKGROUND OF ANOTHER.

PIN TINS

Level of difficulty: ***-*****

MATERIALS: Variety of sea shells, empty 3 1/2 ounce tobacco cans with lids (about 4 1/2 inches in diameter), craft glue, brushes, scissors, solid fabric scraps, decorative braid or trim, varnish or craft glaze (optional), pencil.

APPLICATIONS: Sea shells hold a fascination for men, women, and children alike. All will enjoy arranging shells. Try exchanging stories of past trips to beaches. Sell the completed cans as pin tins for dressers. The faint odor of tobacco remains as a pleasant aroma whenever the box is opened.

PREPARATION BEFORE CRAFT SESSION: Wash and dry the tobacco cans. Place a lid on a piece of plain fabric. Trace a circle around the lid and cut it out. Brush the top of the lid with glue and place the circle of fabric on it. Then brush the side of the lid with glue and place braid or decorative trim completely around the circumference of the lid. The lid should now be neatly covered so that its original design does not show.

CRAFT SESSION: Pick out about 24 medium size shells and glue them in place. Keep adding shells until all crevices are filled and the shells are piled high. For an attractive effect, place some shells upside down or on their side edges. If you like, paint the finished lid with varnish or commercially available craft glaze. Be sure to do this away from patients, as the fumes may be harmful. Note that buttons may be substituted for shells.

PIN TINS

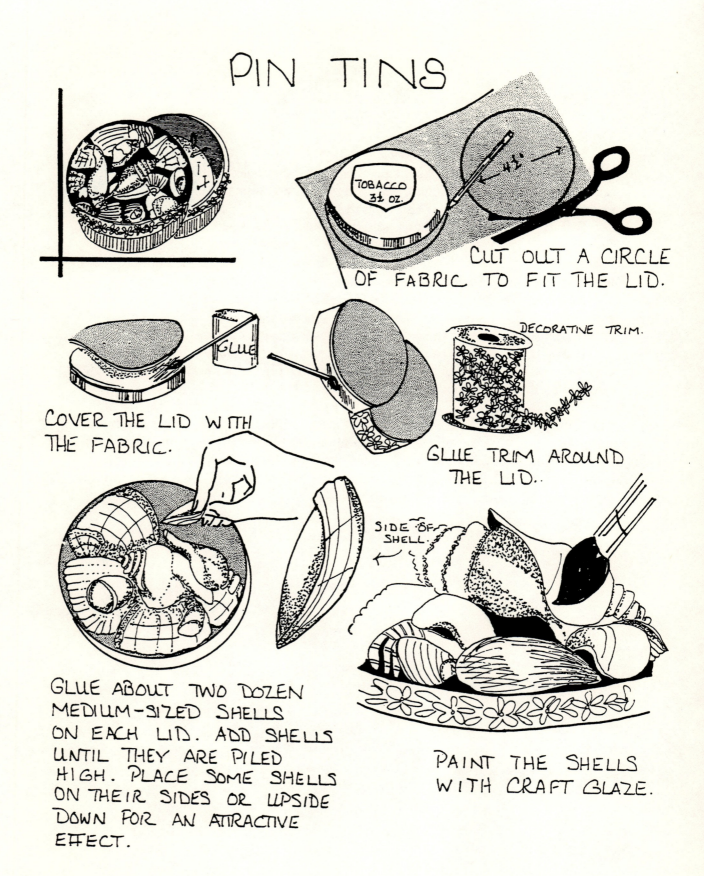

CUT OUT A CIRCLE OF FABRIC TO FIT THE LID.

TOBACCO 3¼ OZ.

COVER THE LID WITH THE FABRIC.

GLUE

DECORATIVE TRIM.

GLUE TRIM AROUND THE LID.

SIDE OF SHELL.

GLUE ABOUT TWO DOZEN MEDIUM-SIZED SHELLS ON EACH LID. ADD SHELLS UNTIL THEY ARE PILED HIGH. PLACE SOME SHELLS ON THEIR SIDES OR UPSIDE DOWN FOR AN ATTRACTIVE EFFECT.

PAINT THE SHELLS WITH CRAFT GLAZE.

DECORATIVE BOXES

Level of difficulty: *-*****

MATERIALS: Cigar boxes, craft glue, brush, spring clothespins, scissors, unbleached muslin or felt or paint, dominoes, nuts, bolts, washers.

APPLICATIONS: The clothespin box is attractive enough to become a decorative coffee table box. Try displaying it open and filled with a notepad, pencils, tape, and scissors. Show the domino box filled with cards and scorecards or children's game parts. And show the nuts and bolts box filled with men's accessories.

PREPARATION BEFORE CRAFT SESSION: Cover the cigar boxes with fabric or felt or paint them a solid neutral color. Be sure to cover the insides, too. Remove the springs from the clothespins.

CRAFT SESSION: Choose clothespins, dominoes, or nuts, bolts, and washers to cover a box. Brush glue on the box, a section at a time. Cover the entire box with the decorative objects.

DECORATIVE BOXES

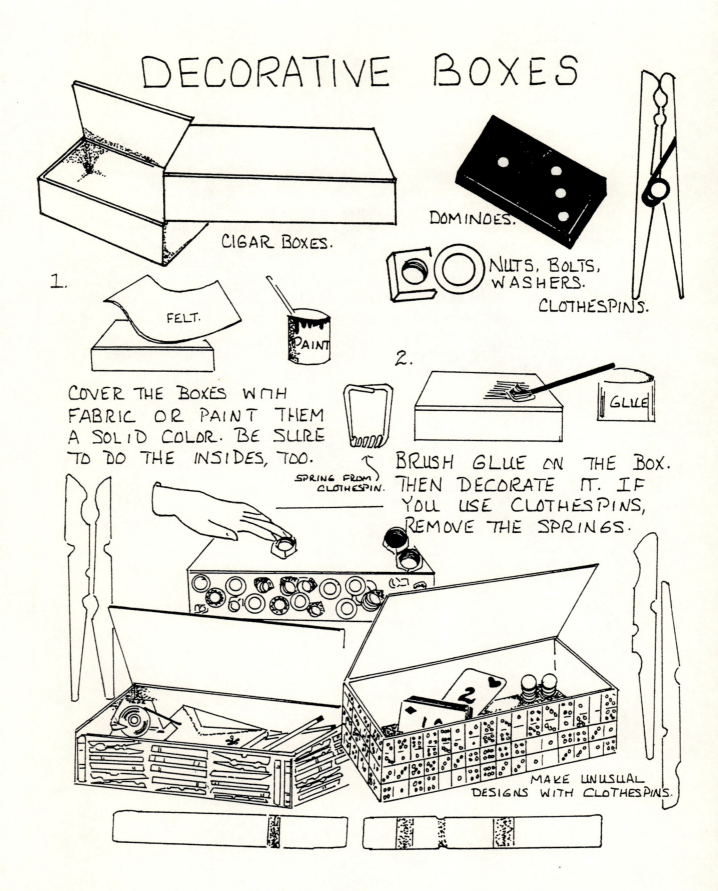

CIGAR BOXES.

DOMINOES.

NUTS, BOLTS, WASHERS.

CLOTHESPINS.

1.

FELT.

PAINT

COVER THE BOXES WITH FABRIC OR PAINT THEM A SOLID COLOR. BE SURE TO DO THE INSIDES, TOO.

SPRING FROM CLOTHESPIN.

2.

GLUE

BRUSH GLUE ON THE BOX. THEN DECORATE IT. IF YOU USE CLOTHESPINS, REMOVE THE SPRINGS.

MAKE UNUSUAL DESIGNS WITH CLOTHESPINS.

WALL HANGINGS

Level of difficulty: ***-*****

MATERIALS: Pink, red, and green felt, scissors, craft glue, brush, heavy cardboard, watermelon seeds, ric rac.

APPLICATIONS: Any kitchen would be brightened by one of these wall hangings. Be creative and make other fruits and vegetables.

PREPARATION BEFORE CRAFT SESSION: Wash and dry some watermelon seeds (a great excuse for a watermelon party). Cut cardboard 6 inches by 9 inches. Cut pink felt 6 inches by 9 inches. Follow the pattern of illustration and cut out the green rind and red watermelon.

CRAFT SESSION: Brush the cardboard with glue. Cover it with pink felt. Glue the green felt on the center of the covered cardboard. Glue the red felt on the center of the green felt. Glue watermelon seeds on the red felt. Trim the wall hanging with ric rac placed about 1/2 inch from the borders.

WALL HANGINGS

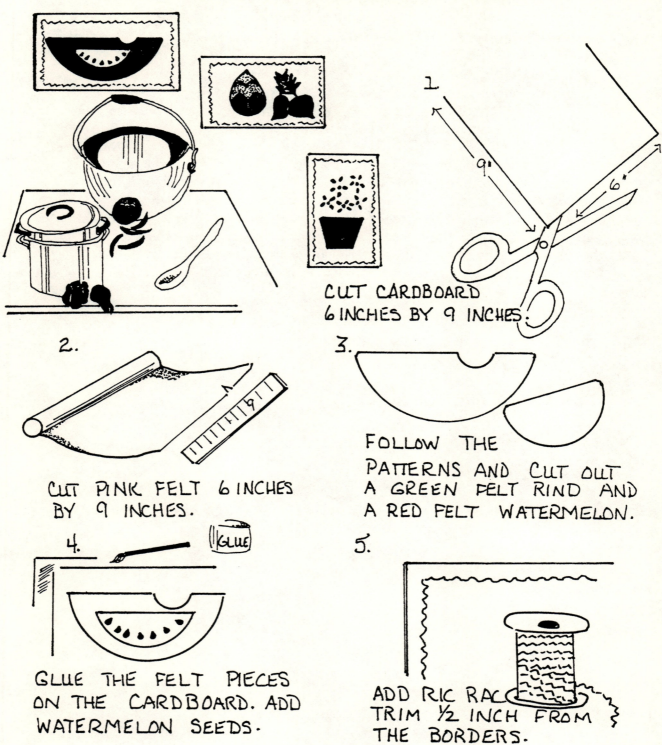

1. CUT CARDBOARD 6 INCHES BY 9 INCHES.

2. CUT PINK FELT 6 INCHES BY 9 INCHES.

3. FOLLOW THE PATTERNS AND CUT OUT A GREEN FELT RIND AND A RED FELT WATERMELON.

4. GLUE THE FELT PIECES ON THE CARDBOARD. ADD WATERMELON SEEDS.

5. ADD RIC RAC TRIM ½ INCH FROM THE BORDERS.

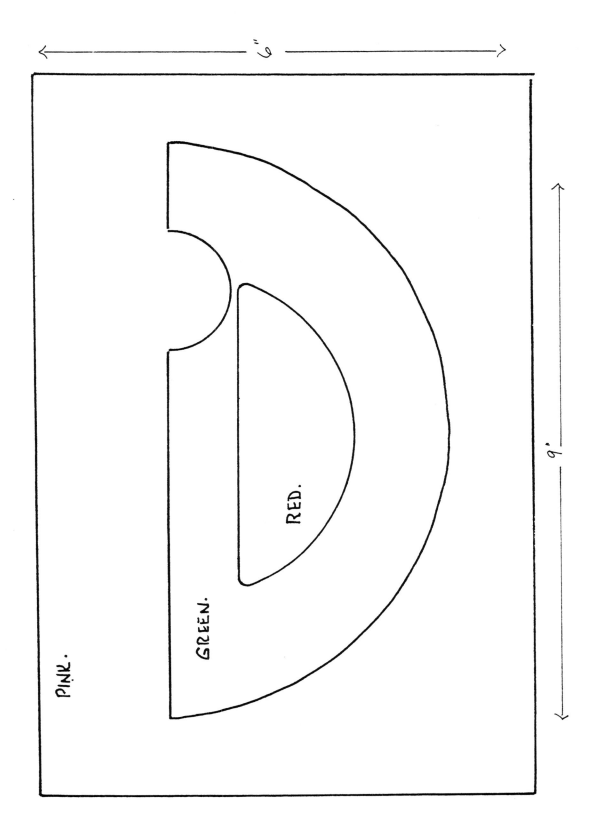

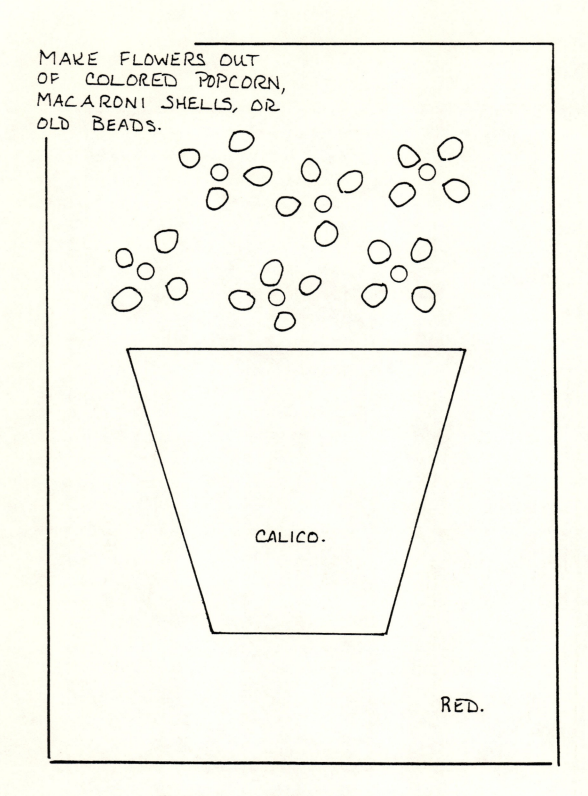

MAKE FLOWERS OUT
OF COLORED POPCORN,
MACARONI SHELLS, OR
OLD BEADS.

CALICO.

RED.

PATTERN FOR WALL HANGINGS.

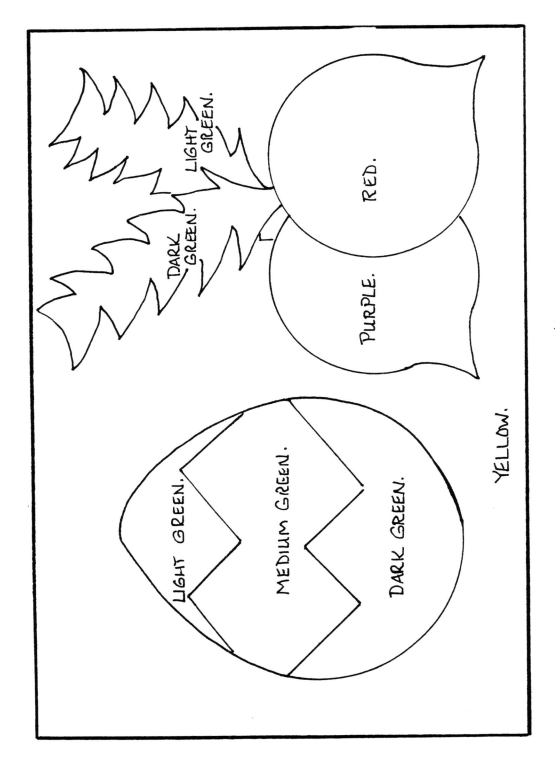

LIGHT GREEN.

DARK GREEN.

RED.

PURPLE.

LIGHT GREEN.

MEDIUM GREEN.

DARK GREEN.

YELLOW.

PATTERN FOR WALL HANGINGS.

STRAWBERRIES

Level of difficulty: *****

MATERIALS: Walnuts, green felt, scissors, small screw eyes, black felt marking pens, gold metallic cord, empty plastic produce baskets, tissue paper, red water-base paint, string, coat hangers, newspapers.

APPLICATIONS: Summer is a good time to make these pretty berry necklaces. If you have a free source for walnuts, make lots of strawberries and arrange them in a basket to sell as table decorations. You may even want to cover the basket with cellophane and tie a pretty bow around it.

PREPARATION BEFORE CRAFT SESSION: Carefully insert a screw eye in one end of each walnut. Cut out one large and one small leaf for each walnut out of green felt.

CRAFT SESSION: Attach one end of a piece of string to a coat hanger. Run the other end of the string through several screw eyes on the walnuts. Then attach this end to the coat hanger. Now dip the walnuts in the red paint and hang them over newspaper to dry. Each individual walnut can be painted with a brush or cotton swab, but hands do get messy. When the nuts are dry, cut the string and remove and save the screw eyes. Place the small leaf on top of the large leaf. Attach the leaves to the walnut by screwing a screw eye through the centers of the leaves at one end of the nut. Then using a black marking pen, make dots all over the painted nut. Run a long piece of gold cord through the screw eye and tie a knot. Make some to fit adults and some to fit children. Display them nicely on a piece of tissue in an empty plastic produce basket.

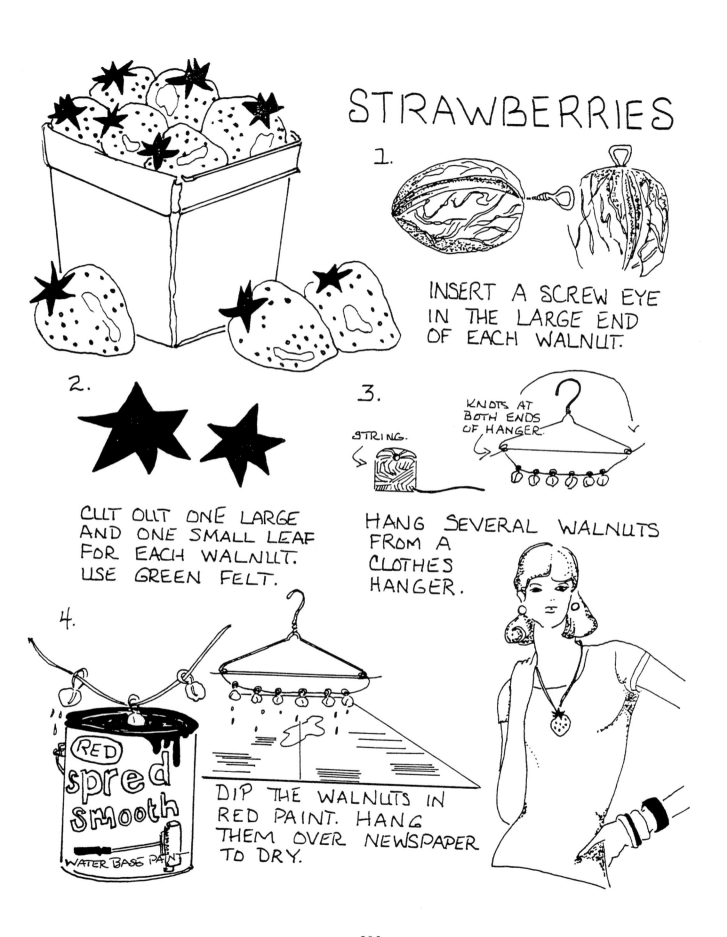

STRAWBERRIES

1.

INSERT A SCREW EYE IN THE LARGE END OF EACH WALNUT.

2.

CUT OUT ONE LARGE AND ONE SMALL LEAF FOR EACH WALNUT. USE GREEN FELT.

3.

STRING.

KNOTS AT BOTH ENDS OF HANGER.

HANG SEVERAL WALNUTS FROM A CLOTHES HANGER.

4.

RED spred smooth
WATER BASE PAINT

DIP THE WALNUTS IN RED PAINT. HANG THEM OVER NEWSPAPER TO DRY.

STRAWBERRIES

5.

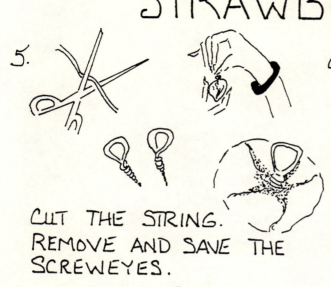

CUT THE STRING. REMOVE AND SAVE THE SCREWEYES.

6.

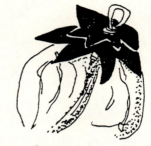

PLACE THE SMALL LEAF ON TOP OF THE LARGE LEAF. ATTACH IT TO THE RED WALNUT WITH A SCREWEYE.

7.

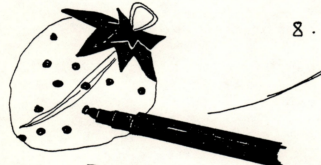

USE A BLACK FELT PEN TO MAKE DOTS ALL OVER THE PAINTED NUT.

8.

TIE A LONG GOLD CORD THROUGH THE SCREWEYE TO MAKE A NECKLACE.

9.

DISPLAY THE NECKLACES ON TISSUE IN EMPTY PLASTIC PRODUCE BASKETS. OR MAKE LOTS OF BERRIES FOR A TABLE DECORATION.

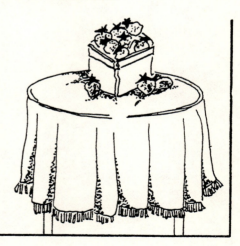

CHRISTMAS ANGELS

Level of difficulty: ****-*****

MATERIALS: Spring clothespins, fabric scraps, net, glitter, craft glue, brush, pop-tops, felt marking pens, pinking shears, scissors, metallic thread, empty margarine tubs, newspaper.

APPLICATIONS: These little angels are practically costless to make and priceless in appeal. Make dozens and cover a tree with them. They will sell themselves.

PREPARATION BEFORE CRAFT SESSION: Follow the pattern in the illustration and using a pinking shears, cut out skirts. Cut out strips of net 12 inches by 6 inches. Cut pieces of metallic thread 12-inches long. Put glitter in one margarine tub and glue in another.

CRAFT SESSION: Draw a face, hair, collar, and hands on the clothespin. You may want to do this on both sides of the clothespin. Dip the 12-inch sides of the net into glue and then into glitter. Shake the net over newspaper to remove the excess glitter. Choose a skirt for the bottom of the clothespin. Secure it with glue. Do this by brushing glue on the clothespin. You may want to dress both sides of the angel. Make a fan out of the net or gather it together in the center and insert it under the spring of the clothespin. Now fan out the wings. Put a loop of thread through the top of the clothespin. Finally, put a pop-top through the angel's head and bend it forward to create a halo. The spring will hold the halo in place. Insert two pop-tops back to back if you are dressing both sides of the angel.

CHRISTMAS ANGELS

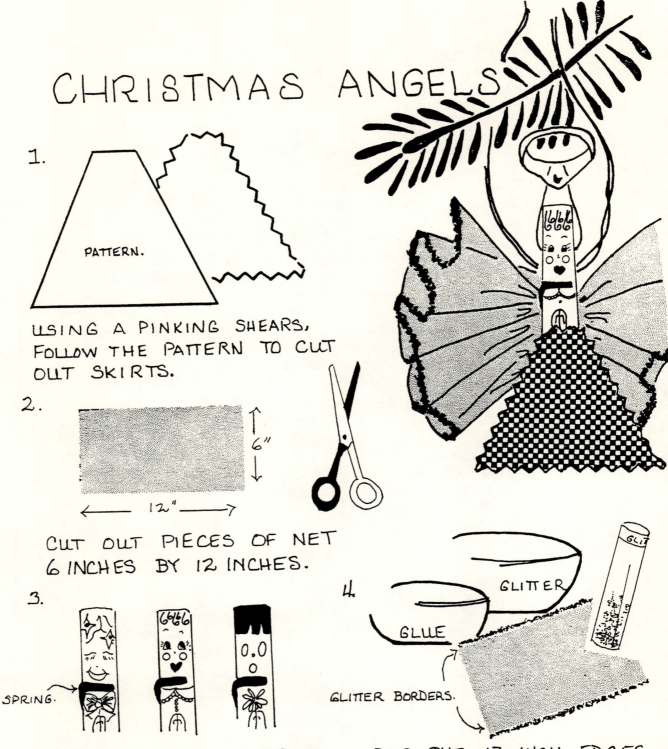

1. USING A PINKING SHEARS, FOLLOW THE PATTERN TO CUT OUT SKIRTS.

PATTERN.

2. CUT OUT PIECES OF NET 6 INCHES BY 12 INCHES.

6"

12"

3. USE FELT PENS TO DRAW FACES, HANDS, COLLARS, AND HAIR ON CLOTHESPINS.

SPRING.

4. DIP THE 12 INCH EDGES OF THE NET INTO GLUE AND THEN INTO GLITTER.

GLITTER

GLUE

GLITTER BORDERS.

CHRISTMAS ANGELS

5.

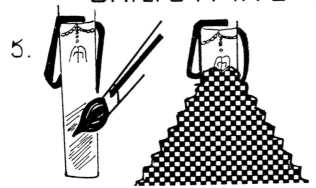

BRUSH GLUE ON THE BOTTOM
OF A CLOTHESPIN AND
ATTACH A SKIRT.

6.

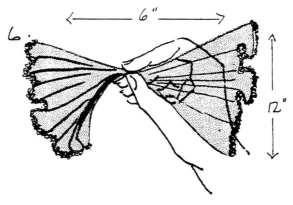

6"

12"

GATHER THE NET
IN THE CENTER.

7.

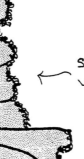

SIDE
VIEWS.

INSERT THE GATHERED
NET UNDER THE SPRING
OF THE CLOTHESPIN.

8.

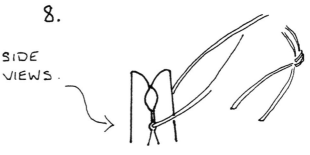

TIE A 12 INCH LOOP OF
METALLIC THREAD THROUGH
THE TOP OF THE CLOTHESPIN.

9.

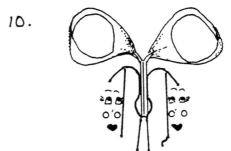

POP TOP
REMOVED FROM
SODA CAN.

PUT A POP TOP THROUGH
THE TOP OF THE ANGEL'S
HEAD. BEND IT FORWARD
TO CREATE A HALO.

10.

FOR EXTRA ATTRACTIVENESS,
DECORATE BOTH SIDES OF
THE ANGEL. ONE PAIR OF
WINGS IS ENOUGH.

WHEAT HOLDERS

Level of difficulty: ****-*****

MATERIALS: One cup salt, two cups flour, one cup water, putty or kitchen knife, decorative twine or yarn, rolling pin, cookie sheet, cooking oil, varnish or craft glaze, brush, wheat or dried weeds or straw flowers, oven, self-hardening clay (optional).

APPLICATIONS: These dainty wall vases add a nice flavor of nature to any room. A grouping of several vases is especially appealing. If you have a gift shop, hang some on the wall for an attractive display.

PREPARATION BEFORE CRAFT SESSION: Prepare dough by combining flour and salt in a bowl and mixing well. Add water, a little at a time, mixing as you pour to form a ball. Knead seven to ten minutes until dough is smooth and firm. Oil the cookie sheet.

CRAFT SESSION: Use a rolling pin to roll out dough about 3/8 inch thick. Cut an oval out about 5 inches long by 2 1/2 inches wide. It does not have to be symmetrical. Then cut out a rectangle of dough about 2 1/2 inches wide by 3 1/2 inches long. Lay one finger over the oval as shown in the illustration. Cover that finger with the rectangle of dough. Using the other hand, press the side edges of the rectangle onto the oval. Be certain to moisten all connecting surfaces so that they will bond. Leave the top open. Remove the finger by sliding the hand downward. Then connect the bottom section. Make a small hole in the center of the top of the holder. Bake the completed holder at 325 degrees for 1 hour and 30 minutes or until hard. Let it cool and then coat with varnish or craft glaze. Use an odor free glaze, if you are glazing in the session around patients. Tie a pretty loop through the hole and insert several pieces of wheat or flowers. You may use self-hardening clay, if you do not have access to an oven.

WHEAT HOLDERS

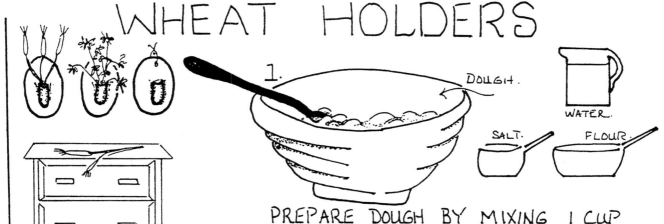

1. PREPARE DOUGH BY MIXING 1 CUP OF SALT, 2 CUPS OF FLOUR, AND ONE CUP OF WATER. KNEAD THE DOUGH 7 TO 10 MINUTES UNTIL IT IS SMOOTH AND FIRM.

2.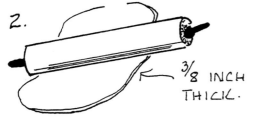

3/8 INCH THICK.

USE A ROLLING PIN TO ROLL THE DOUGH.

3.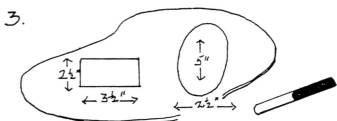

CUT AN OVAL AND A RECTANGLE OUT OF DOUGH.

4.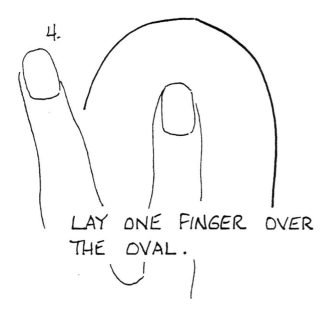

LAY ONE FINGER OVER THE OVAL.

5.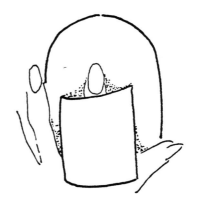

COVER THAT FINGER WITH THE RECTANGLE OF DOUGH.

WHEAT HOLDERS

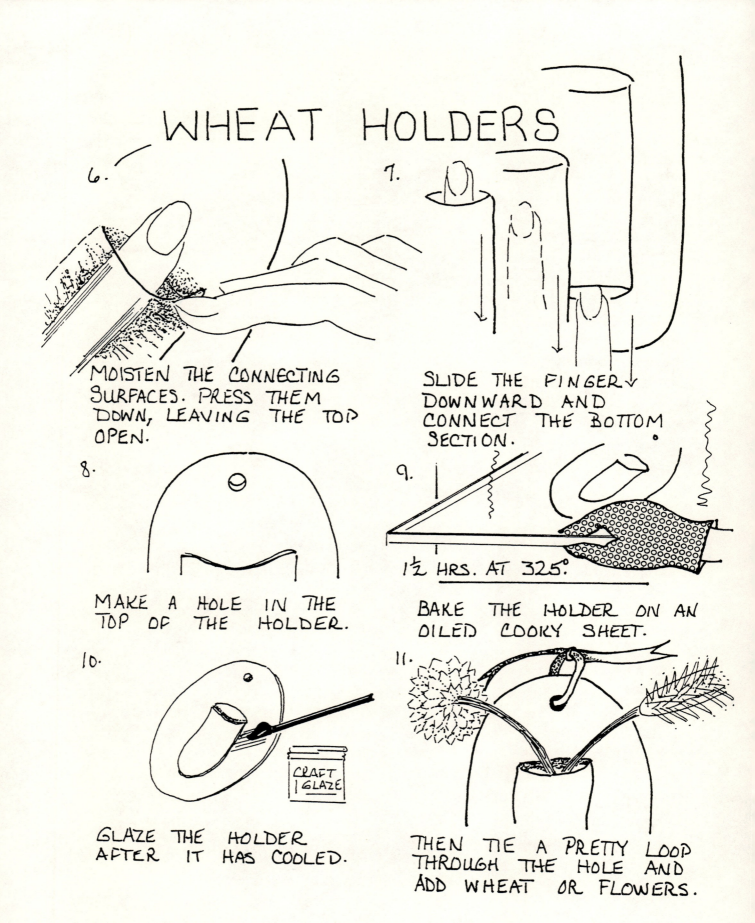

6. MOISTEN THE CONNECTING SURFACES. PRESS THEM DOWN, LEAVING THE TOP OPEN.

7. SLIDE THE FINGER DOWNWARD AND CONNECT THE BOTTOM SECTION.

8. MAKE A HOLE IN THE TOP OF THE HOLDER.

9. 1½ HRS. AT 325°

BAKE THE HOLDER ON AN OILED COOKY SHEET.

10. CRAFT GLAZE

GLAZE THE HOLDER AFTER IT HAS COOLED.

11. THEN TIE A PRETTY LOOP THROUGH THE HOLE AND ADD WHEAT OR FLOWERS.

DECORATED THUMBTACKS

Level of difficulty: *****

MATERIALS: Thumbtacks (red, yellow, white), permanent black marking pen, plastic wrap and cellophane tape.

APPLICATIONS: Neatly done, these tacks make clever, inexpensive gifts that everyone can use for bulletin boards, offices, kitchens, workshops, or stocking stuffers.

PREPARATION BEFORE CRAFT SESSION: None.

CRAFT SESSION: Decorate the red tacks as apples and ladybugs, the yellow tacks as happy faces, and the white tacks as daisies. Be very careful that the ink does not get on clothing. Using the plastic wrap and tape, rewrap the tacks. Put them onto clean corrogated board if necessary.

DECORATED THUMBTACKS

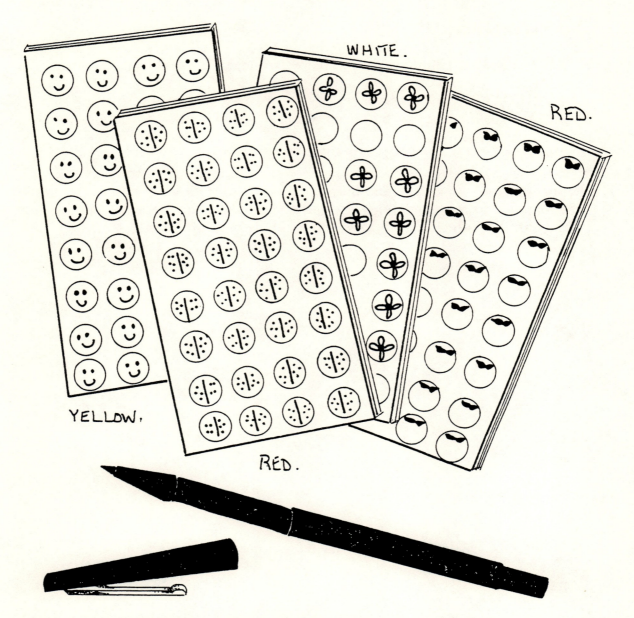

YELLOW.

RED.

WHITE.

RED.

USE A PERMANENT BLACK FELT TIP MARKING
PEN. DECORATE YELLOW TACKS AS HAPPY
FACES, WHITE TACKS AS DAISIES, AND RED
TACKS AS LADYBUGS AND APPLES.

CLOWN CUPCAKE DECORATIONS

Level of difficulty: **

MATERIALS: Wooden ice cream spoons, felt, felt marking pens, glue, scissors.

APPLICATIONS: Package the decorations in half dozen groups, and display them cleverly. Use imagination to make soldiers, patriots, cowboys, Santas, etc.

PREPARATION BEFORE CRAFT SESSION: Using felt pens, draw faces on the spoons. Precut the felt clothing for the decorations. Assemble the necessary felt pieces in front of each person. Leave some spoons without faces for those who like to draw.

CRAFT SESSION: Let those who like to draw design their own faces with felt pens. Then have each person glue the felt clothing onto each spoon. Be careful to leave one half of the spoon empty to be inserted into a cupcake. You could also package these to be used as bookmarks or garden markers.

CUPCAKE DECORATIONS

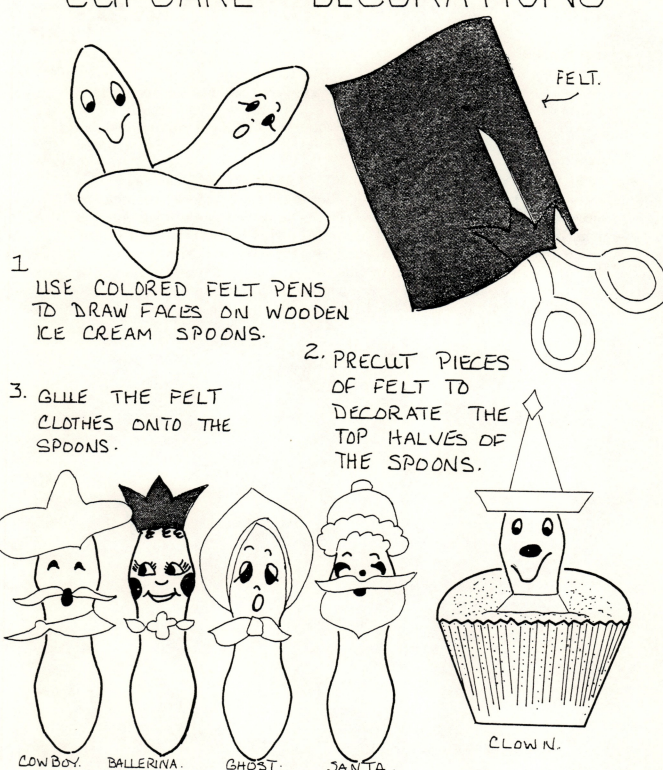

FELT.

1 USE COLORED FELT PENS TO DRAW FACES ON WOODEN ICE CREAM SPOONS.

2. PRECUT PIECES OF FELT TO DECORATE THE TOP HALVES OF THE SPOONS.

3. GLUE THE FELT CLOTHES ONTO THE SPOONS.

COWBOY.   BALLERINA.   GHOST.   SANTA.

CLOWN.

NOTECLIPS

Level of difficulty: *-****

MATERIALS: Spring clothespins, cardboard, felt, colored pipe cleaners, felt marking pens, glue, scissors (ric rac, optional).

APPLICATIONS: These colorful noteclips are clever gifts to sell for any desk or kitchen counter. Clothespins are also useful to keep plastic bags or bread bags tightly closed but easily opened, to attach notes or gasoline receipts to automobile sun visors, and to secure diaper pails bags on car trips.

PREPARATION BEFORE CRAFT SESSION: Cut cardboard and felt the same sizes from patterns, one cardboard and felt pattern for each butterfly and two cardboard and felt patterns for each apple. Cut out dozens of tiny pieces of varied colored felt to decorate the butterflies.

CRAFT SESSION: For the butterfly, draw a happy face with felt pens on the closed end of the clothespin. Then glue the felt to the cardboard and decorate these wings with bits of colored felt and ric rac. Help each person spring the clothespin to slip in the wings and a pipe cleaner for antennae. To make an apple noteclip, glue red felt to the cardboard pattern. Also glue a bit of green pipe cleaner to the back of the cardboard and protruding above the apple to provide a stem. Then glue a felt covered pattern to each side of the clothespin.

NOTECLIPS

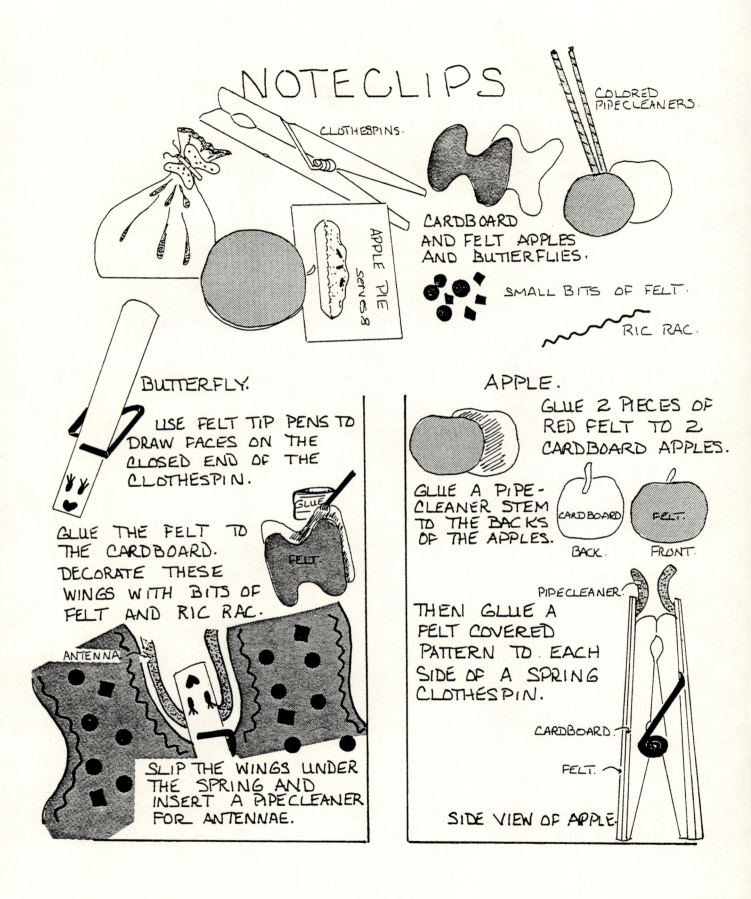

CLOTHESPINS.

COLORED PIPECLEANERS.

CARDBOARD AND FELT APPLES AND BUTTERFLIES.

SMALL BITS OF FELT.

RIC RAC.

APPLE PIE serves 8

BUTTERFLY.

USE FELT TIP PENS TO DRAW FACES ON THE CLOSED END OF THE CLOTHESPIN.

GLUE THE FELT TO THE CARDBOARD. DECORATE THESE WINGS WITH BITS OF FELT AND RIC RAC.

GLUE

FELT

ANTENNA

SLIP THE WINGS UNDER THE SPRING AND INSERT A PIPECLEANER FOR ANTENNAE.

APPLE.

GLUE 2 PIECES OF RED FELT TO 2 CARDBOARD APPLES.

GLUE A PIPE-CLEANER STEM TO THE BACKS OF THE APPLES.

CARDBOARD

FELT.

BACK.

FRONT.

THEN GLUE A FELT COVERED PATTERN TO EACH SIDE OF A SPRING CLOTHESPIN.

PIPECLEANER.

CARDBOARD.

FELT.

SIDE VIEW OF APPLE.

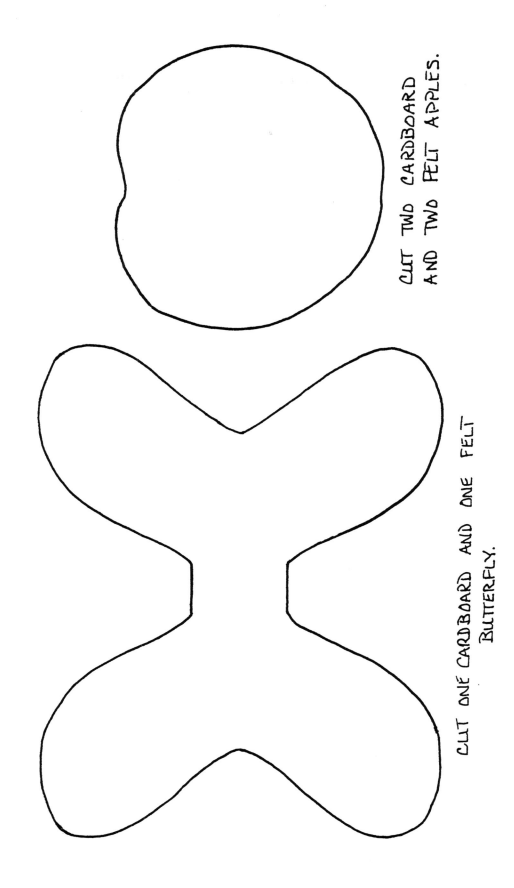

PATTERNS FOR NOTECLIPS

CUT TWO CARDBOARD AND TWO FELT APPLES.

CUT ONE CARDBOARD AND ONE FELT BUTTERFLY.

BIBLIOGRAPHY

Bonner, Charles D. (1974). *Medical care and rehabilitation of the aged and chronically ill.* Boston: Little.

Brocklehurst, J. C. (1973). *Textbook of geriatrics medicine and gerontology.* Edinborough: Churchill Livingstone.

Brook, Peter, Degan, Gian, and Mather, Marcia (1975). Reality orientation, A therapy for psychogeriatric patients: A controlled study. *Br J Psychiatry, 127:* 42–5.

Busse, Ewald W. and Pfiffer, Eric (1973). *Mental illness in later life.* Washington, D.C.: American Psychiatric Association.

Butler, Robert N. (1975). *Why survive? Being old in America.* New York: Har-Row.

Coleman, James C. (1964). *Abnormal psychology and modern life.* Glenview: Scott Foresman.

Cowdry, E. V., and Steinberg, Franz U. (1971). *The care of the geriatric patient.* St. Louis: Mosby.

Cruickshank, William M. (1963). *Psychology of exceptional children and youth.* Englewood Cliffs: Prentice-Hall.

Ferguson, Elizabeth A. (1963). *Social work.* Philadelphia: Lippincott.

Gould, Elaine, and Gould, Loren (1971). *Crafts for the elderly.* Springfield: Thomas.

Harris, Jay, and Joseph, Cliff (1973). *Murals of the mind.* New York: International Universities Press.

Isaacs, Bernard (1973). *An introduction to geriatrics.* Baltimore: Williams & Wilkins.

Jaeger, Dorthea, and Simmons, Leo W. (1970). *The aged ill.* New York: Appleton.

Kessler, Henry H. (1970). *Disability—Determination and evaluation.* Philadelphia: Lea and Febiger, 1970.

Kimmel, Douglas C. (1974). *Adulthood and aging.* New York: Wiley.

Nagi, Saad Z. (1969). *Disability and rehabilitation.* Columbus: Ohio State University Press.

Quiltich, H. Robert (1974). Purposeful activity increased on a geriatrics ward through programmed recreation. *Journal of the American Geriatrics Society, Vol. XXII,* 5:226–29.

Rossman, Isadore (1971). *Clinical Geriatrics.* Philadelphia: Lippincott.

Scott, Louise B., May, Marion E., and Shaw, Mildred S. (1972). *Puppets for all grades.* Dansville: The Instructor Publications, Inc.

Seehafer, Marianne, and Seehafer, Sandra (1974). *Easy crafts for the classroom.* Dansville: The Instructor Publications, Inc.

Sharples, Diana (1993). *The therapeutic arts education.* Stow: Polar Productions.

Simpson, George (1960). *People in families.* New York: Crowell Collier.

Walters, Barbara (1970). *How to talk with practically anybody about practically anything.* Garden City: Doubleday.

Wankelman, Willard F., and Wigg, Philip (1993). *A Handbook of Arts and Crafts (8th Ed.)* Dubuque: Brown and Benchmark.

Willard, Helen S., and Spackman, Clare S. (1971). *Occupational therapy.* Philadelphia: Lippincott.

Wolff, Kurt (1959). *The biological, sociological and psychological aspects of aging.* Springfield: Thomas.